AMAZING
GRACE:
ENJOYING ALZHEIMER'S

AMAZING GRACE:
ENJOYING ALZHEIMER'S

BY
RAY SMITH
AND
ANDREW CROFTS

metro

Published by Metro Publishing Ltd,
3, Bramber Court, 2 Bramber Road,
London W14 9PB, England

www.blake.co.uk

First published in hardback in 2004

ISBN 1 84358 089 6

British Library Cataloguing-in-Publication Data:

A catalogue record for this book is available from the British Library.

Design by www.envydesign.co.uk

Printed in Great Britain by CPD

1 3 5 7 9 10 8 6 4 2

Papers used by Metro Publishing are natural, recyclable products made from
wood grown in sustainable forests. The manufacturing processes conform to the
environmental regulations of the country of origin.

The methods of treating Alzheimer's disease in this book worked for us, and I have no doubt in my mind that they will work for you too. However, I should point out at the outset that I am not a doctor. What I am proposing may be common sense, but it is nevertheless revolutionary. It is important that you should consult a qualified medical practitioner before undertaking any new treatment, or changing any existing one.

FOREWORD

I have been in contact with Ray Smith for over five years. Ray is one of the genuine heroes of our time.

When his beloved wife, Grace, developed Alzheimer's disease, he refused to put her into a home but insisted on caring for her himself. But he did so much more than that. He took her travelling both at home and around the world, going to many places which much younger and more physically able people might have thought difficult.

He looked after her in every possible way and gave her a quality of life which few people at any age can expect. And, by the nature of the disease, he did this without any hope or expectation of return, other than the reward of knowing that she appeared to be happy and to enjoy doing things in his company. Such devotion is not only rare, it is close to unique.

I very much hope that this book will be read widely as an inspiration not only to those who may find themselves in a similarly difficult situation, but to anyone who is captivated by stories of genuine human greatness.

Dr David F. Horrobin

Laxdale Ltd

Dr Horrobin was the eminent scientist who researched nutritional therapy for the mentally ill. He died in April 2003.

PREFACE

The purpose of this book is to show that someone with Alzheimer's disease, or any other disabling illness, can have as good a life as any able-bodied or able-minded person and may, in some instances, even achieve things they never dreamed of when they were fully healthy.

I believe that our whole approach to health and happiness needs to be rethought. Instead of fighting off the side effects of our modern lifestyles with ever-more-complicated chemical concoctions, we need to understand what it is that our bodies actually need in order to thrive. What is it that we are missing that is making us ill? How can we put the good things back into our lives, and help to prevent the illnesses from taking root in the first place?

Of course, some illnesses are inevitable, particularly when

we live the way we do today. When they happen, we need to find ways to make the most of them and enjoy the changes they force in our lives rather than fear them. When illness strikes, the temptation is to shut up shop and close in on oneself. We give up travelling, sex, parties and fun because we think we are too ill for such things. But these are exactly the sort of things that bring health and happiness.

How much better do you feel when you have just laughed long and hard? How much do your spirits lift when everyone around you is smiling? How easy is it to worry about your ailments when you are distracted by new and exciting experiences?

Staying in a darkened room, huddled in blankets and frightened to face the world because we have some physical or mental problem, merely makes the problem worse. By focusing on the things we believe we can't do any more we make those beliefs come true.

I am always struck by the way in which animals cope with disability. If you watch a dog that has lost a leg you will see that it goes about its business with just the same vigour it did when it had all four legs. It may be a little slower, and it may fall over now and again; but it will still be fascinated with every smell, it will still wag its tail and prick up its ears when you speak to it, it will still pursue members of the opposite gender with enthusiasm and eat the same foods it always did with the same eagerness. It simply accepts that one leg has gone and nothing else has changed.

We need to recapture some of that same primitive love of life, and not allow illness and disease to decrease the joy and pleasure that we experience in our lives. We need to be less self-conscious about how we are seen by others, and more willing to risk making fools of ourselves. If it makes you feel good to dance in the streets, then that is what you must do.

It isn't just the victims of illness themselves who need to learn this lesson. Many people feel that, if someone close to them should develop such a terrible condition as Alzheimer's, they wouldn't be able to cope with caring for them. They're daunted by the idea of caring when there might be no respite from the responsibility. They think that, for their loved one's own good, they must dispatch them to an institution where they can receive professional care. They think that by asking someone else to look after their loved one they will somehow be free of the burden and free of the embarrassment of being seen with them in public when they might be making an exhibition of themselves.

But in handing over their responsibility they will have lost that loved one for ever. They may be able to settle down in front of the television for a few hours each evening in peace, but they have no one to chat to and get things for. They may have long nights of uninterrupted sleep, but they will be waking up alone in the mornings, the bed next to them empty and with no prospect of a cuddle or a smile from the person they love the most. Should we only care and protect those who least need our care and protection, those who are in perfect health?

By telling this story I want to show how a loving, supportive relationship can enable both the sick relative and the carer to enjoy an exceptional quality of life, finding new facets of their own personalities, new strengths and new interests as a result of living with the disease.

Caring for Grace was the most rewarding experience I have ever had, giving me as good a life with her as we enjoyed before her illness, possibly even better in some respects. By the end she may not have been the same bright young girl that I married, but what married person can say that their partner of forty or fifty years is unchanged? When you marry someone you vow to stay with them 'for better, for worse', which means that the one who is struck down by ill health must be able to rely on the other not to abandon them. It might have been hard work looking after her, but what relationship isn't hard work in one way or another?

Retirement for many can be a very traumatic experience. The work we choose to do while in our prime can give us a reason for living and a sense of effectiveness that is suddenly lost on the last day of employment. Caring for Grace gave me an overwhelming sense of purpose, especially since I feel I have broken new ground using alternative methods of care, successfully treating the biochemical imbalance associated with Alzheimer's with mega doses of vitamins and minerals, preventing the aggressive and challenging behaviour so characteristic in most sufferers of this unrelenting, progressive, degenerative condition.

Over time, Grace progressed from having a slight problem to needing twenty-four-hour nursing care. She had to be fed, bathed and helped at the toilet; she was unable to speak and almost permanently confined to a wheelchair. But she was never in any pain, nor did she seem to be suffering in any way. We never had to resort to drugs of any sort, apart from the usual antibiotics we all take from time to time to fight the occasional infection. I believed she just needed to be loved and encouraged to have respect for herself as a person. I still believe it after twelve years' experience of nursing her.

I promised Grace I would write this book so that we could pass on our experiences to the many thousands of others who either suffer from similar conditions themselves or who have someone close to them who does. I want to dispel some of the fear that we all feel of dementia striking us or our loved ones, and shed some light on to how we can still lead exciting and satisfying lives whatever cards fate may deal us.

Grace and I have, literally and figuratively, climbed mountains together. I have an evangelical urge to lead as many other people as possible along the same paths that we trod.

ACKNOWLEDGEMENTS

I would like to thank all those who helped and
encouraged Grace in her later years, particularly her cousin
Valerie, whose letters of support from Switzerland meant a
great deal to us. I would like to give a special thank you to
my neighbours, Val and James Daly, who helped so much in
sorting out the mass of material I had accumulated about my
life with Grace and about Alzheimer's, and who put it
into enough order to persuade the publishers to
commission this book.

CONTENTS

A NOTE ABOUT MEASUREMENTS

As you will understand when you read this book, I firmly believe that Grace's courses of vitamin and mineral supplements substantially slowed the progress of Alzheimer's disease in her, and gave her a much happier and more comfortable old age. I have found that the best supplements are made by a company called Solgar. It will be useful for you to understand the way in which the supplements are measured.

IU=International Unit. This is an internationally recognised way of measuring certain substances. It is a quantity of a single substance. The weight of a single international unit will vary from one substance to another.

1,000µg (micrograms)=1mg

1,000mg=1g

Illness is the night-side of life, a more onerous citizenship. Everyone who is born holds dual citizenship, in the kingdom of the well and in the kingdom of the sick. Although we all prefer to use only the good passport, sooner or later each of us is obliged, at least for a spell, to identify ourselves as citizens of the other place.

SUSAN SONTAG FROM THE *NEW YORK REVIEW OF BOOKS*

CHAPTER ONE

LOVE AT FIRST SIGHT

Such a morning it is when love
Leans through geranium windows
And calls with a cockerel's tongue.
LAURIE LEE

Grace Riddle was in the hallway of the nurses' home, standing in the middle of a crowd of other girls reading the notices pinned on to a board when I first saw her. It was 1957, and she had just arrived in London from Scotland, along with three other qualified nurses, to start a midwifery course and they were all trying to work out what they were meant to be doing and where they should be going to do it. Hospitals can be big, daunting places for new staff members, just as they can be for patients and their visitors.

There was an air of excitement and expectation surrounding the group; they were starting out on new lives away from their families and friends in a city full of strangers, with no way of knowing what fate might hold in store for them. They were milling around in the echoing, antiseptic passageway with its shiny lino floors, bare walls and stark lighting, chattering and laughing nervously as they tried to work out how this new institution they had joined functioned. Somehow Grace seemed separate from the others, a still, calm, smiling centre that they could all buzz around without disturbing her tranquillity. I had the impression that she was quietly laughing at the madness of the world around her. She seemed to know more than the rest of them already.

In my memory of that moment, so many years ago, her companions were all dark haired and fairly plain of feature. It made Grace stand out even more with the glow of her blonde hair, pinned neatly up on top of her head, and the fineness of her narrow-boned face and pale skin. Her nose was not small or pert as might be fashionable in young girls, but elegantly, timelessly curved; her blue-grey eyes seemed to sparkle with a mixture of wisdom and mischief. It seemed as if she had already been to places the other girls had never been, as if she had learned some lessons from life and already acquired wisdom beyond her years.

In all truth I cannot say that I analysed the impression that Grace made on me in that corridor at that moment. I was, after all, a young man, and my first thoughts were that Grace was quite simply the most beautiful woman I had ever seen. Nevertheless, the impression remains nearly half a century later, and so it must have imprinted itself on my subconscious at the time. In that first moment, though, and even without the benefit of hindsight, it was clear that Grace was a cut above any of the girls I had ever associated with.

It was love at first sight and first sound. Not only did she look like an angel, but when she spoke she had a low, gentle voice that soothed my soul. Everything she said chimed perfectly with what I thought and believed, confirming opinions I hadn't even realised I held until I heard myself babbling them out to her. When I started to talk to her it was as if I had discovered another part of myself, a better, wiser, warmer part. It was not something I was used to. Out on dates with other girls in the past, I'd struggled to make conversation. I would spend long evenings searching for some common ground, trying to dig up some nugget of information from inside them that might suggest my companion was in possession of some secrets which I might want to find out – all to no avail.

I must have cut something of a frantic figure in Grace's calm, amused eyes. Twenty-seven years old and in my last year of a three-year nursing course at St Giles Hospital, I was a young man with an eccentric appearance and an enormous number of opinions on just about everything. I would cycle around London with my shoulders down over the dropped handlebars of my prized racing bike, my shorts flapping in the wind, desperate to see and do everything that was on offer, pleased to show off my calf muscles to anyone who cared to look. I used to get the women in the kitchens at St Giles (I stayed in the doctors' accommodation at the hospital) to make me up packs of sandwiches on my days off and I would ride down to the coast to resort towns like Southend. I would swim in the sea and eat my lunch on the beach before heading back to the city. The cold salt water would make my skin prickle pleasurably and any shafts of sunlight that I could find would revive me for the return journey. I loved to be out and travelling under my own steam. I loved the feeling of the wind on my bare skin, the scenery speeding past as I pedalled with all my strength, thoughts crowding my head as I concentrated on the road ahead and the pedals under my feet. I would sometimes cover a hundred miles in a day.

I was equally happy with my own company or talking to anyone who sat still long enough for me to strike up a conversation. Shyness was never my problem. I never cared what people thought of me and I was interested in anything anyone had to say to me, young or old.

Trainee nurses received a good number of perks in those days, which helped to make up for the terrible pay. I expect they still do. Theatres and concert halls would give us free tickets in order to fill up their empty front rows with happy, grateful young people. It would make their shows look like sell-outs, encouraging the performers to give of their best. Sometimes I would take my dates to the shows, but more often I would go on my own in order to savour the experience on my own terms. Once I met Grace, however, I never wanted to go to anything without her.

Music, according to Doctor Johnson, is the only sensual pleasure without vice. Grace loved music like I did, and she was happy to talk about anything we went to see together. She was also a wonderful dancer, and tried hard to teach me how to partner her. Eventually, to the regret of both of us, she had to admit that I was a hopeless case and quite likely to trample her to death if she wasn't careful.

Music was by no means our only topic of conversation. We would sit in local pubs, nursing our drinks to make them last as long as possible, just talking and talking – politics, the future of the planet, what life was all about! It would always be the same, right until the end, when it was me having to talk for both of us and she was left with no ability to comprehend anything that I was saying or demonstrate any sort of response. In truth, though, it was probably me doing most of the talking in the beginning as well, because Grace had a knack of making me feel as if she was fascinated by every word I uttered, encouraging me with her enthusiasm to ever greater flights of rhetoric and fantasy. I was full of my own experience, and certain that I knew exactly what should be changed in the world to make it a better place for all of us to live in. She was very good at letting me think that she agreed with every word I said and was fascinated by every idea and thought that I threw at her. And she was brilliant at making you feel you knew everything she was thinking, when in fact she was actually giving virtually nothing away.

If we were going out together, of course, I had to abandon the bike and we resorted to the buses and underground like everyone else, or just to the power of our own legs, wandering around the city, gazing at the sights and ferreting out the nuggets of history that were hidden in every corner. Walking together would always be a big part of our lives, until Grace wasn't able to walk any more.

Even with all the imagination in the world, however, there's a limit to how many things two young people with no money can do together in the city on their day off. 'We could go back to bed,' Grace suggested the first time we found ourselves confronted with a long afternoon, poor weather, no money and no plans.

In my head it was like a giant choir had burst into song, sending hallelujahs soaring thankfully up to the heavens.

After meeting Grace I would never even think of making love to anyone else. I was completely and absolutely in love with the pretty blonde nurse from Scotland with her shy smile and firm, quiet views. No one else could possibly have competed with her and so I never allowed anyone else even to try.

Looking back now at those two young people, pressed together in the single bed in my room, on a floor of the hospital that was meant only for the doctors and male nurses and strictly off-limits to the female staff, I can hardly believe how little I knew about anything. I thought I was so well travelled and so versed in the ways of the world, but Grace had already been through an ordeal of which I was blithely ignorant; the girl who lay beside me had a secret.

I was terrified my new-found joy would slip away as quickly as it had arrived. I didn't know what I had done to deserve such luck; what should I do now to ensure that it continued?

Of course, I was too busy showing off my ideas and ambitions to give too much thought to what might be going on inside the serene head of the woman with whom I was in love.

I was galloping at full tilt with a hundred plans of how I was going to carry Grace along through life with me. The world was still marching to the tired old tunes of post-war austerity. Soon everything would change and I was sure I knew how those changes should be brought about, how life could be made fairer for all and the world made safe and peaceful so that we never had to endure another war like our fathers and grandfathers. They were grand ideas and I was filled with the certainty of youth.

I believe I showed signs of being quite a good nurse once I took the plunge and enrolled for the training. I had to have a job in order to live and I had only the most elementary of educations, so my choices of potential careers were limited. I liked the idea of working in social services, doing something that actually made a difference to other people's lives, people who needed practical help in some way. Nursing seemed a good first step to gaining the necessary experience and qualifications to move on to other, more varied things.

It was obvious, however, why Grace would be led towards such a caring profession. Any patient would feel safe and comfortable waking up and seeing her serene face bending over them in bed. She would have made them feel as if all her attention was focused on them, as if they were the most important person in the world and the restoration of their health the most important task imaginable.

Nursing is a job that gives you a window on to the extremes of life, if you care to look. While working on the wards you witness the great joys of new babies being brought into the world, the fear of those who realise their bodies or their minds are starting to betray them, and the wonder they experience when they're offered a reprieve. You also see the degradation that can result when frail living tissues begin to wear out and malfunction. You see, every day, the untidy aspects of human existence that most people are able to ignore for most of their lives. You learn not to be afraid.

We are all exposed to illness in ourselves and in others at some stage of our lives, but most of the time we can pretend it doesn't exist or that it is something which will happen to others. We can spend our lives pretending that death is never going to claim us, until the evidence is finally presented before us. Even then we often go on believing there is going to be a last-minute reprieve, like in one of those old movies where the man wrongly imprisoned on death row is granted a pardon, just as he sets out on his final walk.

Nurses cannot do that. They are surrounded by evidence of our mortality every hour of their working day and so, in some ways, they have a greater grasp on the realities of life than other people. In the course of their daily routine, nurses can see their own past and a range of possible futures on display in their patients.

In the hustle and bustle of the wards, among the sluices where the bedpans were hosed down, I gave such matters little thought, just taking one day at a time and coping with each problem as it arose. For me it was a living and it would do until I was qualified to take up some better way of supporting myself.

Nursing gave both Grace and me very pragmatic attitudes to life and death and the illnesses that sometimes come along the way. We tended not to dwell on the misfortunes of life, just getting on with sorting them out in the best way we could. It was an attitude that would stand us in good stead later, when it would have been all too easy to give in to despair.

As you grow older it's tempting to envy the young and to forget just how hard youth can sometimes be, not knowing what lies ahead and trying to make your way in a world that seems to be determined to put every obstacle in your path. At times I was almost overwhelmed by excitement at the thought of what might lie in store for me in the coming years, and then fearful that none of it would happen and life would end up being no more than a drudge, as I had seen it become for other members of my family. I was determined that, whatever happened, I would have as interesting a time and as much fun as it was possible to have in my short stay on earth.

I might have been only twenty-seven, but I had already been out of school for nearly half those years. When I reached fourteen, my father told me to get out into the world and start to earn a living and find my feet. No one in our family was that interested in the idea of an education, so the thought of staying on to study further, possibly even going to university, didn't even come up. My father worked for Baker Perkins Engineering, which was one of the main employers in the Peterborough area where I was born and schooled. He called himself an engineer, but I think he was really an unskilled labourer. He was perfectly happy with his life and saw no reason why I shouldn't be similarly satisfied by whatever sort of work I might fall into.

I was their second son, but when my mother fell pregnant with me my paternal grandmother announced that she would take over looking after my older brother Bill in order to give my mother more time for the new baby. I'm sure in those days it was not unusual for the grandmothers to help young mothers out in that way, but Bill never really came back home, even once I was no longer a baby. He stayed with my grandmother even after my younger brother, Reg, was born, and shared a bed with our uncle who still lived at home with his mother, having been invalided out of the war with minor mental problems. My grandmother seemed to be satisfied with having one boy in her house because she didn't insist on removing me from home in the same way when my mother was pregnant again. Maybe she just wanted someone to be company for our uncle.

Reg and I would see Bill quite often because my grandmother only lived a few doors away in Milton Road, but he was more like a cousin to us than a brother. It was all very friendly without being intimate. None of us questioned the situation; it was just the way things were. Children didn't question things much in the 1930s. We simply accepted what adults did and what they told us and got on with it.

Our grandmother was a powerful woman. She owned a grocery shop and had enough money to have been able to set up both her sons with their own houses in the same terrace as her, although my uncle didn't want to live in his, preferring the comforts of the maternal home. I have strong memories of her at Christmas. She would invite Reg and me round to see the tree once she had decorated it. It was a splendid sight with all its candles flickering. Peterborough is not far from Grantham, the town where another grocer was bringing up another tough lady called Margaret Roberts, later to become the infamous Lady Thatcher.

My grandfather was a local farmer and had died when my father was just eight years old. He'd been quite a bit older than his wife, I believe, and suffered from a stroke while out shooting, and was brought back to the farmhouse on a cart. Family whispers told me that before he died there was some problem with a business partner who took all his grain, but there still seemed to be enough money when the farmhouse was sold for my grandmother to set herself up in business and buy the houses in Milton Road. She was remarried by the time I came along, to a man whom I believe had debts and had to be supported by his wife. I never really understood what had happened; I only knew that my grandmother had a firm hold of the reins of power within the family. None of that toughness or business sense seemed to have rubbed off on my father or his brother, both of whom liked the easy life.

My younger brother, Reg, kept up his studying a bit longer than Bill and me, going on to learn book-keeping before becoming involved with the Jehovah's Witnesses and spending the majority of his life trudging from door to door, spreading the 'message'. In 1975 the leaders of the sect issued instructions that all the Witnesses should sell their homes and head for the hills as the end of the world was approaching. Reg did as he was told, but the months passed and the world continued to turn and the price of property continued to rise, meaning that Reg was never able to get back on to the property ladder. To this day he lives in a caravan with his wife Irene, who is ten years older than him. They were both very kind to Grace and me, many years later, when we came back to Peterborough from our travels and were in need of help.

Bill still lives in Peterborough too, and I did go to see him as well when we returned, but he didn't answer my knock so I left him in peace. We were never what you might call a close family.

Our maternal grandfather was a carpenter, joiner and undertaker. His wife had already died by the time I was born, after having given birth to ten children. Our mother used to take us to the house, which he shared with what seemed liked an awful lot of cats, for the occasional visit. I remember being sick in his sink, but little else! He seemed a kindly man, but he too died when I was only four or five.

Our mother never went out to work, always being there for us in our modest terraced house should we need her. I suspect she lived in fear of her mother-in-law and saw her life's work as looking after my father and us. As a result, Reg and I had a pleasant childhood, going everywhere together, keeping rabbits and chickens, which would later come in handy during the war when meat went on ration.

When his mother died and left him a bit of money, our father gave up work at the engineering firm and bought himself a Ford 8 car to take us out on jaunts around the countryside. I guess that was where the gypsy part of my character stemmed from, always wanting to be on the move, seeing and experiencing new things. In 1936 owning a car was a rarity for people of modest circumstances and I loved the sense of freedom that came from driving out on the almost empty roads with Dad behind the wheel and new exciting sights flashing past the windows.

We would visit zoos, go to the seaside and look at interesting old buildings and other attractions, but mainly our dad liked to go to pubs and drink Guinness, leaving us to our own devices outside. In those days no one worried much about drinking and driving, although I do remember him being taken to court on one occasion after clipping someone else's car. When the war started it became impossible to get petrol for pleasure driving and the car had to go. Our father then went back to work as a security man at a nearby factory. I guess by then he'd finished whatever money he had inherited.

I felt a twinge of envy for the children from my class who went on to secondary school, but it simply wasn't a consideration in our family. My father put more value on his practical ability to build a table than on any book skills. He once proudly carved a weather vane in the shape of a fox – nose to the front, tail behind. There was no alternative on offer for me but to start earning a living as soon as school finished; but doing what? I had absolutely no idea how I wanted to spend my life.

My mother already had a plan as to how to launch me into adult life, taking me along to Barber's the Builders the day after I came out of school. Mr Barber was a contact of her late father and she asked him to give me an apprenticeship. He must have taken me on out of kindness because the war was just ending and there wasn't much work around for building firms in our area, with no one having any money and everyone having other priorities in life beyond extending or improving their houses.

People continued dying, of course, and I remember helping make the odd coffin, slitting the wood so that it would bend to accommodate the corpse's shoulders, and lining the inside with pitch. It was pleasant working around the stove, which stoked up well on cold days, with the pot of glue bubbling on top, but when I saw a job offering more money I was off, delivering papers for WHSmith at East Station, then on to a local auctioneers to help at house sales and the cattle market. Each job was interesting enough for a short time, but the gypsy spirit that my father had instilled in us on our drives around the country was nagging at the back of my mind all the time.

Staying in Peterborough all their lives might be all right for other members of the family, but I had an itch to see more of the world. I had enjoyed the few forays I had made out on my own already.

I had started out on my independent adventures when I was fifteen. Having saved up enough money from my job for a ticket and a week's bed and board, I took a train to Matlock in Derbyshire. Arriving in a strange town with no idea where I would be laying my head that night or what might happen to me before bedtime was very exciting. In my search for somewhere to stay I'd walked halfway up the hill from the station when I fell into conversation with an old lady, Madame Minette, who was standing on her doorstep, arms folded, watching the world go by. She told me she was a performer and singer, which seemed interesting. Behind her I could hear the shrieking of her pet cockatoo as we talked by the open door. I asked if she had a room I could rent and she agreed to put me up for the week and give me an evening meal; she'd even got hold of some cream, a luxury I'd never tasted before.

Having found myself a base, I travelled to Chesterfield the following day to look at the sights, and at the end of the afternoon I asked a policeman the way back to the station. He obviously thought I was too young to be wandering around the country on my own and took me back to the police station, where I was given a large mug of tea and a bun while they contacted my parents to check that it was all right for me to be out and about. Once they'd satisfied themselves that I wasn't a runaway and that my parents weren't remotely concerned for my safety, they directed me to the train station so that I could get back to Madame Minette's in time for tea.

Such modest travel experiences confirmed my opinion that the world was an interesting and congenial place through which to stroll, and that most people would respond with kindness and friendliness if you spoke to them or asked for advice. I never suffered from the sort of shyness or nervousness that so often afflicts teenagers, and my inquisitiveness and enthusiasm for everything new that I discovered overcame any self-consciousness that my youth and ignorance might have imbued in me. I dare say I was rather a cocky young man.

All my travels, however, were limited to England. I didn't know much about foreign parts, other than what I had heard from men who had served abroad in the wars or read in the newspapers that I had delivered for WHSmith, but I was pretty sure there was a great deal to do and see if I could just find a way of supporting myself in the process. People like us, however, didn't get to go abroad unless we joined the forces as international travel was still only for the very rich. It would be many years before the idea of the package holiday would take off.

At last I had a direction to go in and a goal to aim for. I would join the Navy and see the world. As soon as I turned seventeen I volunteered for the Royal Navy and was given a job in vittling, which meant looking after the rum, the food, the clothing and anything else that the sailors might need from the stores in the course of a voyage. In those days there were class divisions even in the distribution of the rum. Petty officers were allowed a tot a day, but the ratings had to have it watered down, which seemed very unfair to me.

I joined a sloop called the *Pelican*, a small diesel-powered warship that set off for the Mediterranean on the Haifa Patrol, capturing Jewish immigrant ships that were illegally heading back towards Palestine. Some of the ships in which the illegal immigrants were travelling were horribly unseaworthy, just like the sort of craft that carry refugees across dangerous seas today when they are willing to risk anything rather than stay in countries where they have been persecuted or allowed to starve. Our job was to intercept them and take them to Cyprus where there were internment camps waiting to hold them while the politicians of the world argued over the future of Palestine.

I loved being out on the open seas and often used to take my hammock out from the cramped, stuffy conditions below deck and sling it from the gun turret so that I could sleep beneath the stars in the warm, fresh Mediterranean air, away from the smell of diesel oil. The other sailors told me that I slept so soundly they actually let the gun off one night without waking me. Sometimes I didn't even bother with the hammock and just settled down on a coil of rope.

In the heat of Haifa a few of us went ashore and some of the more experienced sailors led us into a warehouse filled with fresh oranges waiting to be exported. After years of rationing and shortages in England it was like tasting the nectar of the gods as we pulled back the peel and sucked out the sweet juice. We just walked out with crates full of the succulent fruit and nobody bothered to stop us. There seemed to be very little law enforcement in the docks in those days, and people appeared to be able to get away with just about anything if they had the nerve.

Being in the stores made me pretty popular with the crew and life was sweet in the warmth of the Mediterranean sun as we sailed past the spectacular coastlines of Portugal, Spain, the South of France and Italy, which in the coming decades would grow into some of Europe's most popular tourist playgrounds. Whenever we put into a port most of the other sailors were primarily interested in drinking, but my appetites for more cultural adventures had already been whetted by my father and his trips out in the Ford 8. At one stop, for instance, I went on the road to Damascus, hitch-hiking my way up into the mountains from Beirut in order to enjoy the spectacular views and immerse myself in the history of the area. In Tunis I went in search of a Roman camp I'd read about. I was in no hurry to travel back to the grey skies of England and in Malta I heard of a vacancy for a stores assistant in the Navy base. I applied to stay there for a while and was accepted, but I soon realised I preferred being on the move and arranged to have myself put on another ship, a cruiser called *Euryalus*.

Other appetites were also beginning to nag at my brain and I found that being ashore in a smart naval uniform with a cap, blue trousers, jacket, collar and tie – known as a 'square rig' – acted as a wonderful ice-breaker with the opposite sex. The sort of girls who would never have given a gauche young man like me a second look back home in my civvies were more than willing to respond to an approach from a dashing young man in uniform. I suspect they sometimes thought I was an officer because of the smartness of the outfit.

When the *Pelican* put in at Nice, in the South of France, I met a pleasant French girl called Michelle in a bar. She told me she was the daughter of a schoolteacher and took me back to her flat, allowing me to make love to her with the radio playing music in the background. As far as my memory can tell, that was probably my first time. I think I had made the odd attempt before I left England to persuade girls to let me go a little further than light petting, but with limited success. For a young boy from Peterborough, making love to a French girl in the South of France was a heady experience.

I would happily have stayed in that little flat for the rest of my life, just enjoying the sensual pleasures of music and love, but I had to get back to the ship as we were on our way to Malta. When I finally managed to tear myself away from her arms I practically skipped all the way to the docks, reliving the previous few hours in my mind a hundred times. I wrote Michelle several letters from the base in Malta and laid excited plans for going back to visit her the moment I had some leave.

When I had enough leave saved up to make the trip worthwhile, I bought a boat ticket from Malta to Sicily and booked a train ticket to take me all the way through Italy to Nice. I was about to set out on this journey, knowing it was bound to take at least three days, when I had another idea, which I thought would save me some precious time. I went down to Luca Airport to see if I could hitch a flight with anyone. Other sailors had told me about how easy it was to do.

There weren't as many planes there as I had expected and I was on the verge of abandoning the plan when a Blue Airlines plane came in from Kenya, carrying a coffee magnate to London. I struck up a conversation with him while he waited for the plane to be refuelled and he offered me a seat for the next leg of the trip, but I had to make up my mind there and then as they were about to take off again. I already knew there was no one else offering a flight to France, but didn't know if another flight would arrive at any moment which would whisk me straight to Michelle in Nice. Now I had to choose between a definite free ride home to England to see my family or hanging on in the hope that someone else would come along and offer a ride to Nice and that Michelle would still be there when I arrived. I decided to take the bird in the hand and head for London.

As a serving sailor I didn't need a passport – just showing my pay book was enough to get me over any borders. The coffee magnate sat at the back of the plane, and fooled around with the air stewardess all the way. I sat at the front, keeping my eyes facing firmly forward.

My family were very surprised to have me turning up on the doorstep after about eighteen months away, and I spent a pleasant two weeks at home before realising that I didn't have any guaranteed way of getting back to Malta in time to report for duty. I went down to Heathrow Airport and tried to hitch a ride back in the same way I had come, but failed. The idea of young sailors hitching rides on planes was a great deal more frowned upon in the organised chill of Heathrow than in the casual sunshine of Malta. Instead of being offered a seat going south, I was picked up by the police and escorted to Chatham Barracks, where I had to stay until they managed to find a boat to take me back to face my punishment, which consisted of having no leave at all for some time.

Even though I had heard nothing from her, my experience with Michelle in Nice continued to play on my mind and when

I was next back in England a year or two later I decided to use fourteen days' leave to hitch down to the South of France to surprise her and see if I could pick up where I had left off. I made it all the way down, wearing my uniform to assist with the getting of lifts, which was strictly against the regulations, and managed to find my way to her front door. I rang the bell with my heart thumping, not knowing if she would even be living there any more but secretly dreaming of jumping straight back into bed and taking up where I had left off.

When she opened the door she looked very startled and quickly had to recover herself, inviting me in and explaining that since we last met she had got married to a captain in the French Navy. I was very disappointed, after such a long journey and having rehearsed our passionate reunion so many times in my head, and not a little embarrassed. After some polite but stilted conversation I made my excuses and left.

Like most young men with no regular partner, sex was nearly always on my mind. Some of my fellow sailors, of course, didn't bother to wait until women were available. There were stewards on board who were known as 'officers' bum boys', and old seamen would sometimes take younger men and boy seamen under their wings (thus earning the nickname 'wingers') and look after them. I remember a sick-berth attendant who was known as Queenie and was a complete cabaret act in himself. It was all treated as a laugh but I never got involved myself, my mind being constantly on the girls. Looking back now I think that even then I was hunting for someone who would be my partner and soul mate as well as my sexual collaborator. Right from the start I was looking for Grace, although I didn't realise it until the day I found her.

CHAPTER TWO

Sailor Sacked for a Song

One thing alone I charge you. As you live,
believe in life! Always human beings will live and
progress to greater and broader life.

W. E. B. DUBOIS

Before I left school, a teacher called Mr Anderson managed to trigger my interest in left-wing politics. In those days it was still easy to see the differences between the haves and the have-nots, and there was a class system in place that still made it very hard for people from backgrounds like mine to improve their lot in life and make a mark in the world.

These were the days when Communism in Russia was still looking like a great and brave experiment, before any of the cracks in the system had started to show, and when the benefits of socialism such as the National Health Service and welfare state were being widely debated as the way forward to a more just and equal society. Even as a boy I could see so much that needed changing and had a great deal of hope that, if we kept speaking up about the injustices of the system, life in England could eventually be very different.

It seemed to me patently obvious that the world was an unfair place and that it was the duty of all of us to try to make it more egalitarian. Everyone in my family at that time, however, was true blue Conservative, like much of the traditional working class in those days, so I wasn't able to find anyone with whom I could share my views. I was a bit of an oddball in more ways than one.

Once I started travelling around the world in the Navy, I saw poverty on a far greater scale than anything I'd ever witnessed in Peterborough or other English towns. We might have lived in a modest terraced house with an outside toilet and an old tin bath that you filled from hot kettles, but that was nothing compared to some of the living conditions I saw around the docks that we put into in Europe, the Middle East and Northern Africa. The seeds of socialism that Mr Anderson had sown in my fertile young mind grew at a ferocious rate in the warm sun of other countries. I could see that many of the problems in the world were caused by war and aggression and I began to think seriously about the need for disarmament and the aims of the peace movement.

As long as I was at sea, or based in Malta, there wasn't much I could do apart from think about the things I saw and listen to the other men talking. When I was eventually stationed at an airbase near Oxford, however, I was able to start organising myself to be more active politically, getting ready to play my part in making things better. I could see that being in the forces wasn't exactly compatible with a growing belief in the rightness of communism and disarmament, but I needed the job and I was working hard to follow my conscience whenever I wasn't on duty. Young men with no money have to be practical with their ideals. Quite what I would have done if we had declared war on Russia while I was signed up, I don't know.

Just because I was now no longer at sea, I didn't intend to stop my travelling either. Whenever I had free time I was making plans. There were so many things I still wanted to see and experience. I was particularly keen to peep behind the Iron Curtain, believing that I would find a promised land there, a workers' paradise just like the communist party talked about in all their propaganda.

Deciding that I would only get there if I made the effort myself, I got myself to Hanover and caught a plane from there to Tempelhof Airport in West Berlin. There was no other way into the city other than flying because it was completely surrounded and cut off by the Eastern bloc. It was an exciting prospect for a young communist. Once in Berlin I found myself a boarding house where I could leave my stuff and set off to cross the border into the Eastern sector. I was dressed in civilian clothes as I boarded an underground train, which I knew ran from the Western sector to the Eastern. I disembarked in the Russian zone as if it was the most normal thing in the world to do and made my way towards the ticket barrier, filled with curiosity about what I might see once I wandered out into the fresh air of the 'workers' paradise'.

Before I could get anywhere near the exit an armed policeman swooped on me and ordered me in German to come with him. He led me into a room where other armed guards were congregating, emptying their pistols into a sand bucket before settling down for a break on the spartan furniture provided.

They must have realised quite quickly that I was not a spy of any sort and gave me a chunk of bread and a cup of tea. I'd joined the peace movement in England by that time, and thought that this was a wonderful experience, seeing for myself that the 'enemy', as we were being led to believe the Russians now were, were human beings just like us. I felt that their friendliness towards me vindicated my belief that this was a much better system to be living under than the old imperialism of home, the imperialism that I was happily serving by being in the Navy. Life seemed so full of conflicting interests and needs.

They put me in a cell with some Russian soldiers to sleep for the night and the next day I was interviewed by two Russians who were interested to hear about how I was stationed at Oxford and a member of the Peace Movement. Maybe they thought they had a potential spy on their hands. They had a car and offered to give me a guided tour of the zone, introducing me to some university students, including one very pretty Russian girl, and proudly showing me the splendid new blocks of flats they were building for workers and students alike. It all seemed extremely pleasant and strengthened still further my belief that things back home had to change.

At the end of my propaganda day they put me back on the train to return to the Western zone. After a few minutes, as we trundled through the tunnels, I noticed that one of the other passengers seemed to be watching me with undue attention. I was pretty sure that he had been put there to follow me and, not feeling ready to be recruited for any undercover work on their behalf, decided to lose him by dodging through a few streets before finally going back to my hotel.

It had been an enjoyable trip and so, once I was back in Oxford, I contacted the local paper in Peterborough and told them the story, which they were happy to publish, giving me my first little taste of the limelight. I liked the feeling of seeing my name in print. It seemed to confirm that I existed, not only in my own head, but in the eyes of others as well, and that I was already living a life that was a little out of the ordinary.

Back in England I soon became fidgety once more and started to publicise my political views more widely to anyone who was willing to listen. I enjoyed stirring things up. Like many idealistic young people at the time I subscribed to left-wing magazines and even wrote a song, which I set to the music of the hymn 'Stand Up, Stand Up for Jesus'. I circulated it amongst my colleagues in the Navy until our superiors decided it was rather too revolutionary for a man supposedly enlisted to fight for the English way of life. I could see their point. As far as I remember the song went something like:

> Sign on, sign on for ever
> Ye sailors of the Queen.

Suppress the colonial people
With bayonets, bombs and guns.
Ignore their cries for freedom
Self-government, liberty.
Give all your life for capital
And profits willingly.

I believe there were a couple more verses along similar lines that were passed around until it came to rest in the hands of the officers.

I would also order forty or so copies of the *Daily Worker*, the communist newspaper, and sell it to my fellow workers around the base, making a bit of money at the same time as spreading the word. I was beginning to get a better idea where I was going in life.

I had met a girl on a peace march called Dorothy Hargreaves, whose father was a very left-wing headmaster in Manchester, and he encouraged me to become even more active in the communist cause. On one occasion I travelled to a concert being given by the Vienna Boys' Choir in order to sell newspapers to the crowds outside. It wasn't long before the authorities came to hear about my expanding activities and I was thrown out of the Navy, having served six of the seven years I had signed up for. Marked down as 'unsuitable', I was discharged.

On the day I came out of the Navy I was in Chatham. They equipped me with a civilian suit and sent me on my way with a few pounds in my pocket. I hadn't particularly wanted to leave, but I wasn't too worried by the turn of events either. Coming back to the outside world with all my newly acquired experience seemed like a good opportunity for a new adventure. I made my way to the station to catch a train to London, on my way home to Peterborough. As I walked down the platform, glancing in through the windows of the carriages in the hope of finding a spare seat amongst congenial-looking people, I noticed an ecclesiastical man sitting alone in a compartment. His face looked familiar and I realised it was Dr Hewlitt Johnson, the Dean of Canterbury, who, at the time, was notorious for his left-wing views. His picture frequently appeared in the papers, captioned 'the Red Dean of Canterbury'. I had often read about him in the *Daily Worker*.

I climbed on to the train and walked back to his compartment, sliding open the door that he had firmly closed and letting myself in. I was aware that he had spread his books and papers out on the other seats in the hope of being able to travel undisturbed, but I wasn't going to let that put me off the possibility of meeting such a stimulating travelling companion. Having settled down opposite him I introduced myself and explained what had happened to me. Initially, I dare say, he wished I would leave him in peace to work, but my tale seemed to catch his attention and he suggested that once I reached London I should go to the offices of the *Daily Worker* and tell them my story.

I did as he suggested, finding a sympathetic journalist who wrote down everything I told him and promised to see what he could do. The next day I appeared on the front page under the headline 'Sailor Sacked for a Song'. I was surprised by how easy it was to get your name into the news and pleased to see that my removal from the Navy had had some beneficial effect in spreading the word. Surely it couldn't be long now before I was leading a successful revolution against the might of the tired old British Empire.

Being on the front page of a paper, however, doesn't put food on the table, so I headed back to Peterborough and got a job in the office at Perkins Diesel, where my father and brother had taken jobs after the war, while I thought about what I might like to do next in my grand plan to overthrow capitalism and end war forever.

Even in an engineering firm in Peterborough it wasn't long before my mouth got me into trouble again. I succeeded in offending someone in the office by criticising people who had escaped from the Eastern bloc, the place I still saw as the workers' paradise, and I was fired again. It seemed that someone who had a relative who was a political refugee from communism had heard my naïve and idealistic proclamations and had taken exception to them.

The Communist Party then found me a job at Vauxhall Motors for a year or so but it was just a job and the work I was asked to undertake didn't seem to me to be of any particular use to my fellow man. I still couldn't think how to earn a living while also being of help to people. It was then that my headmaster friend from Manchester suggested I should train as a State Registered Nurse.

The idea instantly appealed to me and I couldn't think why I hadn't thought of it before. Maybe it was because nursing was a profession that was still almost exclusively female. The idea of working amongst so many young women was an added bonus – as well it might have been for a young man with no ties. I applied to St Giles Hospital in Camberwell. I was accepted for training and headed for London with all its sights and excitements. I was almost the only man on the course and it was a pleasant experience being surrounded by so many girls!

Being in the big city, however, I was able to explore other interests, particularly music. I didn't know much about classical music, but I knew I liked composers such as Beethoven and Mozart. The seeds of my love for music, which had been sown while I was still in school and used to go to concerts in Peterborough Cathedral on Sundays, had firmly taken root. Because I had been a member of the local Guild of St Peter Youth Club I could sit in the choir stalls of the cathedral for nothing and listen to visiting orchestras. London gave me the opportunity to broaden my musical interests.

As a nurse I was quite good at my job, but that was all it was. I couldn't pretend that nursing was really a vocation for me, but the fact that it led me to Grace means that I couldn't possibly regret any of the decisions I made during those early years. When a male nurse on another course told me that he was going on to university once he had finished his training in order to do social studies, I thought that sounded like a logical step forward.

While I was training at St Giles in Camberwell, and bicycling around the south-east of England, Grace had been training in Scotland. She was five years younger than me and had come down south to London to take a course in midwifery. I can't imagine what my life would have been like if I had not taken the decision to go into nursing and had not chosen to apply to that particular hospital. Although we never know what alternative fates might have awaited us had we taken different decisions in life, I am quite convinced that had I not met Grace I would inevitably have missed out on the greatest experience of my life.

CHAPTER THREE

Grace's Secret

A man falls in love through his eyes,
a woman through her ears.
WOODROW WYATT

Grace's father was an engineer by training, but he had worked as a chauffeur in a well-known biscuit company for most of Grace's childhood. He'd also been to America to work on a ranch, which was when Grace's older sister Helen was born. The whole family had a deep love of animals and her father had looked after horses in the First World War.

Her mother didn't work full-time, although I think she did sometimes take part-time jobs as a waitress. Both her parents had great compassion for the common man and her mother had taken part in the campaign to allow Paul Robeson, the black singer and political activist, to be allowed to leave America and travel the world with his act. Because of her parents' interests and backgrounds she understood many of the things that I believed in, and didn't look at me as if I was some madman when I started holding forth on my various hobby horses, as most other girls I had met had done. We had so much to talk about, so much we wanted to find out about one another. When you've been with someone for fifty years it is hard to believe that there was ever a time when you knew nothing about them and they knew nothing about you.

I guess a chauffeur doesn't earn much, and it seemed to me from her descriptions of her childhood that her family was fairly poor – although some of the time had been spent living in a grand house in Edinburgh that they had looked after for her father's employers while they were away. Grace had left school at about the same age as me and done a few mundane jobs before deciding on nursing. Like me she was the middle child, with a younger brother, Robert, as well as her older sister.

Although she didn't talk about it much, my impression was that Grace hadn't got on particularly well with her mother. She had become ill after Grace was born and so as a small baby she had been looked after by her grandmother for the first couple of years, which seemed to mean that mother and daughter had never really bonded properly. It also meant that she understood how things were in my family, with my grandmother bringing up my brother, without having to ask. We both had many shared experiences, and often we simply understood one another without having to say anything. Although we talked all the time, we seldom touched on the more personal questions.

As she grew up, Grace was seen by her family as being a bit

of a rebel, hanging out with the wrong sort of people and going to the wrong sort of places. In those days teenagers had to do very little in order to earn a reputation for being wild. Her nickname within the family was 'Turk'. Her father, the main breadwinner, had died of cancer a few years before I met Grace, and making ends meet was obviously a terrible struggle for those who were left behind.

Grace and I had so much in common. She was interested in the peace movement, just as I was, and her father had been a reader of the *Daily Worker*. We went together to demonstrations in Trafalgar Square and to concerts at the Festival Hall. We explored everything that London had to offer that wouldn't cost us any money.

Whenever I wasn't with Grace, I would be writing pages and pages of poetry to her, for her and about her. She had completely bowled me over, making me unable to think about anything else for more than a few minutes at a time before my mind would wander back to picturing her.

The worst moments of the day for me were when she had to leave my room after making love in order to return to the female nurses' quarters. After so much warmth and togetherness, excitement and pleasure, the stark room felt devastatingly silent and empty. The moment the door closed behind her I could think of nothing else but her; I could still smell the scent of her hair on the pillow.

As long as I was writing my poetry to her I felt we were still together, still connected in some way, and I was able to get through the loneliness and keep all other thoughts at bay by scribbling frantically until I eventually fell asleep. In the morning I would wake up thinking about her and would hardly be able to wait until I got down to the wards and saw her again, proudly handing over the sheets and sheets of writing I had done for her. Every day was the same. She filled every nook and cranny of my world.

While being in love is a wonderful experience in many ways, it is also a terrible burden and a curb on a young man's freedom to behave however he chooses. Until I met Grace I had never been frightened of losing anything or anyone. I had been able to do or say whatever I wanted whenever I wanted. To be honest, I didn't have anything to lose, and there is a great freedom in that situation, particularly when you are young and don't realise what you are missing by not having someone to love. Suddenly, with the arrival of Grace in my life, I was worried that she might go off me, or someone else might come along with more to offer and steal her away. I was constantly frightened that it was all going to end; certain that I would never again be able to find someone who would make me feel the way she did; certain I would be unable to live a happy, productive life without her.

Other people in the hospital must have known what was going on between us since I was glued to her side at every possible opportunity. Because my room was in the doctors' quarters there was a lady who came round to make our beds and tidy up for us. One day I came back to find she had made the bed as usual and neatly laid out two discarded condom packets on the bedside table, which I must have lost in the bedclothes somewhere the night before. If the authorities knew we were flouting the rules, they chose not to say anything and we were allowed to continue as discreetly as possible.

However good the social life might have been, Grace and her friends from Scotland didn't like the working atmosphere at St Giles Hospital and she didn't finish the midwifery course, moving on instead to a job as a sister at a geriatric hospital in Lewisham, an area just next to Camberwell. I have to admit St Giles wasn't an inspiring place at that time and I was keen to find something else myself. I was anxious, though, not to be parted from Grace for a moment longer than was necessary in any day.

She rented herself a flat in Finchley Road, close to Swiss Cottage underground station on the north side of London. I also left St Giles and got a job in another geriatric hospital while I finished off my qualifications for social work.

One of Grace's greatest qualities was her sphinx-like ability to be discreet and to keep a secret. If she didn't want to share something that was going on in her head she was able to hide all clues of its existence. I had no idea that she was harbouring a secret during the early months of our relationship. While I gushed out every detail of my life, she was withholding something that must have taken up a large proportion of her thoughts, even when she was in my arms.

We had been going out for several months before she told me about the existence of Anne, her daughter, who had been born after Grace accidentally fell pregnant at the age of fifteen, just after leaving school. There had been clues to Anne's existence, but I hadn't chosen to piece them together, happy to take Grace completely at face value. I'd seen a picture of a pretty little girl on the mantelpiece in her flat and she'd casually told me it was a relative's child. In those days there was still a great deal of stigma attached to children conceived out of wedlock. She might have been frightened that I would leave her if I knew she had a daughter, or she might just have got so into the habit of discretion that it had become second nature to her. She certainly needn't have worried. There was nothing in the world she could have told me that would have made me think less of her. My love for her was completely overwhelming and a small thing like an accidental teenage pregnancy and a daughter in Scotland did not make the slightest difference. I was quite sure that I would be able to love any child of Grace's, whoever the father might be.

I didn't insist on knowing the details of what had happened, but she told me anyway. Anne's father was a taxi driver who had been about twice her age at the time and, apparently, had got himself into similar scrapes before. There was no question of them marrying when the pregnancy was discovered and so Grace's family had rallied around her. Anne was being looked after by Grace's Auntie Rena while Grace found her feet in the world and acquired a profession that could support them both if necessary. Rena, Grace told me, had never had children herself, having married an American who turned out to have a wife in every port, and she had never met anyone else.

I looked forward to meeting Anne as soon as we had enough money for a couple of tickets back to Scotland.

Like many young men, I guess I was pretty self-centred about the relationship. I was so contented with our life together, my head so busy with my own plans, that I hadn't really given any thought to how Grace might like our lives to progress. Even though I was terrified of losing her, I didn't think about what I should be doing to make sure I held on to her. I was just hanging on and hoping for the best. I should have been paying more attention.

A German nurse who became a friend of Grace's had a boyfriend from Mauritius. The two of them were planning to go around the world on an extended holiday, along with his brother, and they asked Grace to join them. It was obviously a very tempting offer, one I would have been keen to take up myself if I hadn't been so besotted with Grace. When she told me about this invitation, and confessed that she was actually thinking of accepting, I was panic-stricken. I'd been letting our life together jog along nicely, not really thinking that I needed to take decisive action if I wanted to keep hold of her. Now she was considering going off around the world with a complete stranger! This was a shock. In fact it was unthinkable! How could I possibly remain in England, all the time imagining what was happening on a glamorous tropical island on the other side of the world? If Grace had been wanting to galvanise me into action she couldn't have thought of a better way of doing it.

She told me about the planned trip in my room at the hospital, and then left before I could respond. I was just sitting there, my mouth hanging open and my heart thumping hard enough to burst, unable to think what I should be doing to save the situation. As the door closed behind her I felt the most terrible desolation spread over me, and I knew that I had to do something radical and immediate if I didn't want to lose her forever. The room was so empty without her, I couldn't possibly have coped if I had thought she wasn't coming back. My brain was in complete turmoil.

As usual, unable to keep my thoughts inside my head, I poured them out into a poem, which I gave to her the next day, having spent a sleepless night imagining the horror of having to wave Grace off at the airport as she walked away with another man, and of then living through the following months of torture as I imagined the wonderful experiences she was having, without me there to share them; having to read postcards full of excitement and news while I sat alone in my room. I still have the poem, which reads as follows:

A rose has left my room
The place is gaunt and bare.
The walls which had a cheerful hue,
Are deathly pale for lack of you.
A rose which so much filled my room
Has left and gone; now all is gloom.

With majesty she chose a place
And all around was light and grace.
Her eyes would sparkle, dazzling all

To bow and worship, there befall.
The pictures, paintings turned their heads,
Nymphs and fairies to their beds.

The sun would never dare to shine
Unless by token to your shrine.
I'm mean and helpless, always thine.
Will you, darling, please be mine?
If life and joy together be,
Dearest, will you marry me?

She was used to receiving poems from me in the mornings, and read it with her usual amused little smile. I waited, hardly able to breathe, for her to reach the final line and the all-important question. She seemed to be reading it through several times before answering and for an awful moment I thought she might be playing for time while she thought up a way of letting me down lightly. I studied every flicker of her expression, trying to work out if I could detect the traces of a frown, or a glint of pleasure, but Grace was always a mistress of discretion and understatement.

Finally she looked up, smiled, nodded and said 'yes'. I could breathe again. All thoughts of her disappearing off around the world with someone else were banished, and I felt safe once more.

The next problem was deciding how best to take this giant step into marriage. Neither of us, nor our families, had enough money to put on a big ceremony and reception, so it was going to have to be the bare minimum. We went to Wood Green Registry Office and I hauled a couple of ladies in off the street to act as our witnesses. Neither of us minded what happened as long as we ended up married. For me, the ceremony passed in a haze of happiness and I can hardly remember a thing about it. I kissed Grace, gave each of the witnesses ten bob for their trouble and the whole thing was over. We had made a commitment to love and honour one another, in sickness and in health, for as long as we both should live. It was a commitment that I knew I would always fulfil, no matter what might happen. It was, and always would be, inconceivable to me that I would ever give up caring for Grace, and I couldn't wait to get started on my new husbandly duties of care and protection.

These were times before anyone had heard of such concepts as 'women's lib'. I saw my role as being Grace's protector and, although fashions changed and Grace sometimes protested at the role she had been allocated in our marriage, I was never able to envisage myself in any other way.

In our travels together around historical London we had taken an interest in everything to do with Dickens. I had heard of a hotel called The Leather Bottle at Rochester which had strong Dickensian connections, and I booked us in there for our wedding night. We travelled over by train after the ceremony. One night was all I could afford, but it was a good one. We had a bottle of champagne and a quiet time together in peaceful surroundings. We didn't need anyone or anything else. At last I felt safe that she was mine and would be until death did us part. It was safe now to turn my mind to other things like making a living and having an interesting and enjoyable life together.

Making a life together in London was always going to be hard for two young people on low salaries. The cost of property was higher than in other parts of the country even then, and there was greater competition for every job. We decided that we would move up to Scotland to set up home there. That way Grace could look after her daughter and we could become a proper family.

We duly handed in our notices and caught the train north. When we arrived I was introduced to Anne, who was a delightful child, and I was delighted to take her on as part of my new little family. To be honest, I was so in love with Grace I wouldn't have minded if she had had ten children and we had had to feed and clothe them all.

There was never any great strife between any of us in those years. Anne seemed happy to call me Dad, but I was never comfortable with the idea of exerting authority over her, not having been involved in the early years of her life. Sometimes Grace would want me to tell her off for something, as a father normally would, but it never felt right. I didn't feel it was my place. Anne's initial bonding had been with Grace's aunt, rather than with us, but we still managed to get on peacefully most of the time.

Now all I had to do was work out how I was going to feed my new family, and what I wanted to do with the rest of my life.

CHAPTER FOUR

BACK ON THE ROAD

There's nothing surer,
The rich get rich and the poor get poorer.
In the meantime, in between time,
Ain't we got fun?
GUS KAHN AND RAYMOND B. EGAN

I enrolled as a mature student at Glasgow University, studying for the Certificate in Social Studies with a view to completing my journey towards becoming a social worker. I was able to get a grant, which was enough to support the three of us in our modest lifestyle – we were living in a couple of fairly basic rooms in a house on the outskirts of Edinburgh. The course was two years long and could lead to a career in social work or possibly even a job in personnel. No doubt I would have earned more money in the personnel department of some big company, but whether my tendency to speak my mind on controversial issues would have sat comfortably with a corporate career, I don't know.

At the university we had lectures on social economics, history, psychology, sociology, politics, law and even philosophy. It was all interesting stuff, which fitted in with the left-wing interests I had been developing since leaving school. Despite my lack of secondary education, I had already developed and fed my insatiable curiosity about the world in which I lived so, if intellectual curiosity is one of the prerequisites for being a good student, I certainly fulfilled that criterion. All my views chimed well with the general feeling amongst my fellow students at the time about social equality and the need to end war.

Grace didn't go back to work once we were in Scotland, wanting to devote as much time as possible to Anne in order to make up for the early years she had missed while in London, and it wasn't long before she became pregnant again. Clifford, our first son, was born in 1960.

From a practical point of view, having another child was not a particularly wise idea, but we weren't very practical people and so we were very excited at the prospect of starting a new adventure with a baby of our own. I built a nursing chair for Grace out of old packing cases. I might not have been as capable with my hands as my father, but necessity was the mother of invention and I was very proud of my achievement.

Once we were four, instead of three, the flat soon became too small for us, so, when I read in the paper that the Scottish Special Housing Association was renting out old miners' cottages at Douglas in Lanarkshire, I applied for one. Although it was about thirty miles out into the country, it was affordable and I could hitchhike in and out of the city for lectures. I enjoyed that sort of lifestyle, being out in the fresh air, meeting different people on the road every day, setting out in the morning with no idea what adventures might lie ahead, taking my chances and relying on my luck.

At last, after all those years in tiny flats and lodging rooms, we had our own little house and it was worth any amount of inconvenience to be able to come home to my own front door, knowing that my wife and children were waiting behind it to welcome me. It must have been hard work for Grace to keep the house running and to put food on the table with the tiny amounts of money we had, but she never complained. She seemed to be unafraid of poverty and confident that we would make it through whatever adversities life might throw at us. Caring for small children came naturally to her. They were, after all, a great deal less demanding and needy than most hospital patients, particularly geriatrics.

Grace was wonderful at creating meals for us from virtually nothing, mixing everything with potatoes or chickweed or whatever came to hand. Mince and potatoes were a particular treat, as were 'stovies' – a popular local dish made from sausages with a lot of fat and onions. Grace would always have enough bread to make me some sort of sandwiches to take with me to lectures. There was another dish called Ling Sole, which she made from mushy split peas. We had a little garden where we grew our own carrots, lettuces and cabbages, and on my way home from lectures I would call at the fish market for cheap herrings. One day they were particularly cheap and it was only once I was in the closed confines of the car in which I had hitched my next lift that I realised why. The driver had some pretty pointed comments to make about the pong.

When we first arrived at the cottage I visited a small wholesaler and stocked up on boxes of currants, raisins and dried fruit, along with small bags of dates, figs, tea and coffee. Grace would make some interesting cakes with the ingredients I provided.

One Christmas, Grace's aunts came to celebrate with us and we gave them each a pack of stockings from Santa. On another visit, her Aunt Ann gave me four shillings and sixpence, just over 22p in modern money, which I used to buy a large chunk of cheese in order to boost our intake of protein.

A friend of Grace's Auntie Rena was a sort of electrician who had a small basement shop in which he sold electrical bric-a-brac. He was an enterprising man and would get his electricity from a street lamp outside the shop. He renovated and gave to us a primitive electric washing machine which worked very well. We also managed to save up for our first television, a second-hand set that cost us £10. It was a lot of money but we were so excited to be able to watch fuzzy black-and-white pictures of acts like the Clyde Valley Stompers in our own home.

We hadn't been in Douglas long before Grace was pregnant again with our second son, Kenneth. Christopher came along a few years later. Family planning was not our strong point, and even with our frugal lifestyle money was getting very tight indeed. If it was impractical for Grace to work when she had two small children to look after, it was completely impossible when she had four, so the making of money was all down to me.

Eventually, I had to admit that we needed to be in a city in order for me to find work and make ends meet, so at the end of my university course we moved into Glasgow and I got a job in childcare, which meant there was a small salary coming in. It was much better than trying to live off the grant alone. I later worked as a social worker for the British Polio Fellowship, earning enough to feed the family and keep a roof over our heads, but little more.

Grace and I were still very active in the Peace Movement, even sometimes taking the children with us on marches to protest outside nuclear plants. On these occasions Grace would often be in charge of the first-aid van. Most of her time would be taken up with caring for the teenage protesters who became overexcited and tore themselves on the barbed wire surrounding the plants as they tried to scale the sinister-looking fences. These were the days when the great philosopher Bertrand Russell was still active in the cause of peace, and when it was still considered to be a fringe activity for eccentrics and students in duffle coats. The great majority of citizens, the generations that had fought in one and sometimes two world wars, were still largely deferential to the politicians and military leaders, and believed that talk of peace was for cowards, traitors and left-wing intellectuals. Looking back now, after all the outcry there was against the recent wars in the Middle East, it is encouraging to see how far we have come since those days in terms of the public voicing its own opinion.

High-minded ideals, however, do not feed families, and money was still in desperately short supply as the appetites of the boys grew larger. In an attempt to get together enough cash one week, I exaggerated my expenses claims at work. I'm not proud of this moral lapse but in my defence I can say that I can't have been very convincing as a fraud because I was immediately found out and sacked yet again. This time, however, I was given three months' money in lieu of notice. For the first time ever we had a little money in the bank and I had a breathing space in which to look around and try to find something that would make us a little more cash, rather than rushing straight into the first low-paid job I was offered. There is an old cliché that says that most people are too busy earning a living to be able to make any money. That was certainly true in my case. The jobs I was qualified to walk straight into were all at the very bottom of the pay range. I needed to buy some time to think about what else I might be good at and to look around at what might be available.

Reading through the appointments pages of the local paper one day I saw an advertisement for a company called Nu-Swift Fire Extinguishers. They were offering a week's course in Morecombe, teaching people how to sell their products, with the promise of high commission on sales once I was trained.

This was a long way from anything I had ever done before, but I had a feeling I might be good at it. I would certainly enjoy doing something so different to social work. Once I got started I discovered I really thrived on the challenge of selling and beating targets. I liked chivvying people into giving me orders, and I liked travelling around from one customer to the next. It appealed to the gypsy in my soul, just as the Navy had. It also involved talking to people, another of my specialities, and the product was something that was actually useful.

My territory was half the centre of Glasgow, which included a great many offices, all of which needed by law to have extinguishers and many of which didn't have any at all. Our sales technique was very dramatic. I was equipped with a portable extinguisher, which I could use for demonstrations, so I would start fires in trays in front of the customers, using lighter fuel, and then put the flames out with a great dramatic show. It was theatre and I had always been a bit of a show-off. I suspect many of them thought I was quite mad and agreed to buy just to get me out of their premises before I burned them down. Whatever the reason, I was very successful at getting orders. It was the right product at the right time, and the market was wide open. It was a relatively easy job to point out to employers that they were breaking the law and then offer to take care of the problem for them. Within a few months I was one of Nu-Swift's top salesmen and our family income had doubled almost overnight. I was even able to get a big order from a bank by going round there over New Year, while all the competition was out celebrating. It wasn't considered to be very good form by the competition, but it seemed like fair game to me. Often I would follow up a sale to a well-to-do firm by going to the partners' big houses in the country and talking them into equipping their homes with extinguishers as well.

It wasn't that we were growing rich, or anything close, but

at least now we could afford to look after ourselves in a decent manner without constantly watching every penny. We were even able to buy a house of our own for the first time, instead of renting. I felt proud that I could now say that I was looking after Grace and the children properly, as I felt a husband, father and provider should do.

On top of the money I earned from my salary and commission, there were also the incentive prizes that I kept winning, like a leather coat for Grace and holidays to places like Rome, Estoril and Tunis. The company would hold special holiday promotions when they awarded points to their salesmen for the number of items they sold. Those with the most points would be awarded a holiday. I would always make sure I had enough points to be able to take Grace with me on any trip, which meant we could experience locations that we could not have afforded for ourselves. My urge to travel just never seemed to abate, and if I could do it with Grace beside me I was completely happy.

Everything takes time in life and as the years go by you slowly discover the things that you are good at and the things that make you happy. More than anything else I loved Grace, and was happiest when I was with her. At the same time I loved to travel and be out and about all day long. Now I also knew that I enjoyed selling and persuading people to buy things. I wasn't certain, however, that I wanted to go on selling fire extinguishers forever. To start with, many of my best customers now had as many of the things as I could persuade them to take, so it was becoming harder to gain big sales. It was also fairly dull selling the same worthy but unexciting product day in and day out – when you've set light to several trays full of lighter fuel every day for a year or so the novelty begins to wear a bit thin. I was trying to think of what sort of job I could do next that would combine all the things I loved and still produce a decent income for the family.

Grace and I were both still very keen on music and art and would go to concerts or exhibitions whenever the opportunity arose. It was after we had been to an art gallery in the centre of Glasgow to see the work of a new young painter called James Harrigan, who used fantastic splashes of colour in almost traditional-style landscapes and still-life paintings, that I had an idea that was to shape the next twenty-five years of our lives.

The art we had seen seemed to me to be exceptionally good, but having talked to the artist I knew that he, like most of his peer group, had great difficulty in selling enough to make a living. It appeared to me that the problem was that the sort of people who might buy such pictures weren't the sort of people who would ever think of visiting an art gallery. Most people never buy paintings and don't know where to go, what to look for or how much they should pay. Galleries can be daunting places and prices are usually pretty high, discouraging ordinary people from making casual purchases. It is a big commitment to agree to buy a painting in a gallery, not knowing what it will look like once you get home and hang it on the wall.

I thought that an artist like James needed to take his work

to the potential customers rather than waiting for them to come to him. If I had sat in a showroom with my fire extinguishers, waiting for people to come in and buy them, I doubt if I would have made any sales at all. I had to go to the potential customers and demonstrate why they should buy. Obviously an artist can't spend all his or her time out on the road, otherwise he or she will never have the time to create the work in the first place. I suggested to James that I would sell the paintings on a sale-or-return basis on his behalf, taking a commission on any sales I might make. Not surprisingly, he was very pleased with the idea, and had a studio full of unsold pictures I could choose from. By that time I had a car, so I took some of his paintings out on the road and started knocking on the doors of wealthy-looking homes.

I was amazed by the result. I sold out almost immediately. This, I decided, was what I would do next, and I bade farewell to the fire extinguisher business. We already had a caravan that we had been using for holidays, so I had plenty of space to carry the stock around, and could broaden my range to include other work. I went to see other artists whose work I liked and made them the same offer. Some of them had small pictures that I could sell for thirty pounds or so, others had paintings worth several thousand pounds. I borrowed some money from my friendly bank manager, who seemed to be able to see the same potential in the market that I did, and who held my house as surety just in case I was completely wrong.

We had a family dog at the time, a mongrel called Shandy, whom we had purchased from a dogs' home for two pounds.

Initially he had been for the boys, but they'd soon lost interest in him, as children so often do with pets. I had taken a great shine to him so I took him out on the road with me for company. We must have been a pretty eccentric spectacle as we made our way around the grander areas of Scotland, particularly the suburbs surrounding Aberdeen where the oil money was and where people were moving into new houses that needed decorating. Shandy enjoyed the life as much as I did, although he occasionally got me into trouble with his amorous ways. I called at the house of the writer Lady Antonia Fraser once, and Shandy took rather too much of a liking to her Labrador bitch, chasing it round the corner and then returning, coupled up behind like a goods train, which didn't help my sales pitch. In fact I think it killed it stone dead. I later heard from an estate agent that the Labrador in question had a reputation for worrying sheep, which had made it unpopular in the area, and as a result Shandy received some notoriety for his brave performance.

One of my clients was a Francophile lawyer living in Rubislaw Den. Whenever Shandy and I arrived at the house I would strike a large Chinese bowl gong in the front hall before turning left into the room where he worked, while Shandy turned right and headed for the kitchen. One day, as the lawyer and I sat talking about art, there was a scream from the kitchen and a flustered housekeeper came running in to inform us that Shandy had just helped himself to two splendid fillet steaks which had been awaiting preparation for a lunch my client had planned with important guests. I had to abandon my sales pitch in order to rush to the local market and replace the meat. That lawyer bought a number of paintings from me over the years, one or two of which ended up being gifted to the Aberdeen Art Gallery on his death.

On another occasion I called at the home of Maitland Mackie, a famous local cattle farmer who had been elevated to the job of Lord Lieutenant of Aberdeenshire. He lived in another grand house in Rubislaw Den, the entrance to the extensive grounds flanked by large stone posts surmounted by equally large stone balls. As I drove through the gates I clipped one of the posts and brought its ball crashing to the ground. Worried about possible legal action, I informed my lawyer friend what had occurred. He told me later that he had dined out for months on the story of the man who had destroyed the lord lieutenant's balls.

Sometimes I would be away for several days at a time, living in the caravan like a gypsy. I would cook my meals on a little Primus stove and at night I would sleep amongst the canvases. Shandy had a baby-beaver-skin coat that I had bought for two pounds at a jumble sale, which he liked to be wrapped up in on cold nights. I had a kettle for boiling water and a bowl to wash in and didn't need much more. I had never been a great one for creature comforts. As long as I had something to eat, somewhere to lay my head and something interesting to think about I was content. If we were near the sea Shandy and I would run in there to freshen up, whatever the weather, returning to the road invigorated and ready to sell.

Although this new lifestyle satisfied my urge to travel, it

inevitably meant that I was separated from Grace much more than I would have liked. It would have been impossible for her to leave the boys on their own on school days, and I certainly couldn't fit all of us into the caravan along with the paintings, even if the boys had been willing to come. Every evening, after making my last house call, I would find a phone box and call home, just to hear Grace's reassuring voice before I went to sleep thinking about her. Although I loved being out on the open road, I still missed her whenever she wasn't beside me.

It wasn't long before word reached reporters that there was a strange-looking man with a mongrel dog wandering up people's front paths with oil paintings under his arms. The *Scotsman* did an article on Scotland's first, and probably only, mobile gallery. The publicity helped to make people more comfortable when I turned up on their doorstep. It was as if I had been given some sort of seal of approval; if a reputable newspaper wrote about me then I must be what I claimed to be, and not some burglar in disguise. After a while, as I gained some regular customers and the business built up, I changed the caravan for a Transit van, which was more practical, easier to drive around the back roads and made me look a little less like a cross between a gypsy and a mad professor on holiday.

I loved the selling aspect of the job, going into people's houses and talking them into trying out the pictures on their walls, taking them out to the caravan or the van and laying out pictures on a piece of velvet for them to look at. No one makes a decision about buying an expensive painting quickly, so I had wonderful opportunities to spend time with different people, finding out about them, their tastes, their families, and talking about the art and about Grace and the children. Often it was the wives who would be in the houses during the day while their husbands were out at work and they had plenty of time to chat with someone who was happy to listen. Wandering around people's houses, drinking coffee, gossiping, trying different paintings in different positions on their walls, attempting to work out what sort of thing they would like – it was a wonderful life.

Now and then I would be aware of a little gentle footwork under the table as I sat chatting to these lonely women, suggesting that they would have been happy for me to follow Shandy's example with the spreading of a little love. I was always very careful to extricate myself from such situations without offending them and risking losing a good customer. Being married to Grace, I never felt the slightest urge to take up any of their offers.

I was amazed by just how much money people were willing to spend on art if they were approached in the right way. I was doing even better than I had been with Nu-Swift and we were soon able to move from Glasgow to a bigger out-of-town house in Bishopbriggs. I'm not sure the business would have worked so well around Edinburgh, where there were a lot of good galleries, but in Glasgow at that time there was very little opportunity for people to buy art. I kept adding new artists to my list until I was representing nearly all the best working Scottish artists, and even some sculptors.

The only area I didn't become involved with was abstract art. Even though Grace liked it, I could never get into it and so tended to be rather dismissive of it. I wish now that I had listened a little more to her views on the subject rather than pooh-poohing them so easily. She was a thoughtful woman and wouldn't have developed a liking for something without good reason. I wish I had taken the trouble to find out a bit more about those reasons, instead of assuming that I was the family art expert and must therefore be right in all my opinions. I realise now that I must have crushed her on more than one occasion on the subject, but she was too kind and polite to put me in my place, letting me continue to strut my stuff as the resident art connoisseur of the family.

Sometimes I would organise an exhibition in a hotel, and then the whole family could come too. I also exhibited at the Royal Highland Show where I eventually had a tent, inside which I erected plywood walls so we could hang the pictures in a more professional way. Clifford was getting bigger by then and was very helpful with erecting the walls. It was always good to do things with the boys and, thinking back now, I guess I didn't become as involved in their lives as I should have done when they were little. The problem was that I was away so much, and when I did get home I was exhausted and only wanted to be with Grace. She and I would take our meals in the morning room, while the boys would often be next door in the television room, left to their own devices. I don't think I was a bad father, although they may very well disagree, but I could have been a better one. It's hard work bringing up children, and I think a lot of men like me are more than happy to hand over the major part of the responsibility to their wives, particularly if their wives are as calm and capable as Grace always was.

Maybe if I had taken more time to get to know the boys, listened to them a little more instead of talking all the time, sought out their company instead of always sitting with Grace, perhaps I would have seen the problems approaching and would have been able to do something to avoid them. But it's always easy to see what you should have done with the benefit of hindsight. At the time I hardly seemed to have the opportunity to draw breath, and there were a thousand other things I wanted to do, places I wanted to visit, ideas I wanted to explore.

I was becoming an established figure in the business, albeit an unconventional one, and I was loving every minute of it. Every year Grace and I would be invited to the opening of the Scottish Royal Academy and would get to meet all the artists and the bankers who supported the Scottish arts. I think other people in the art world must have seen how well I was doing and realised there was an unfulfilled demand for art in the parts of Scotland that I was serving. No one else, as far as I know, went as far as to go out on the road, but, as the years passed, more and more galleries started to open in Glasgow and it became harder to sell door to door. I had to keep thinking of new things to offer people.

As well as contemporary artists I also started to buy and sell older works, like nineteenth-century oil paintings, picking them up at auctions and then driving them around to my existing clients, along with the work of my regular artists. Some of them cost me as much as twelve or fifteen thousand pounds and I was having to ask twenty thousand for them from customers. I was beginning to carry an awful lot of stock one way and another, and the number of customers who could afford my products was dwindling. My bank statements were starting to make uncomfortable reading, but I couldn't think of a way to get back to the position I'd been in when I first set out. I didn't know what else to do. I still loved the life, and so I kept pushing on in the hope that something would change. I could tell that Grace, a woman who never normally questioned any decision I made, was becoming exasperated, but I couldn't see any alternative. I had my blinkers firmly in place.

I tried opening a static gallery in an old church, but it was a disaster. I wasn't comfortable being in one place all the time, prowling around the premises like a caged lion waiting for customers to come in. What I liked was moving around, spending time in the auction rooms in London, New York and Amsterdam with Grace, inspired by all their excitement and beauty, buying pictures that we liked and actually doing the selling to customers. It was a fabulous life, like a dream come true. How could I possibly give it up?

Grace particularly loved Holland, often saying that it felt like a second home as we sat drinking beer in the pubs or wandered along beside the canals. We would buy paintings at Sotheby's and Christie's salerooms and take them back with us. Our flights usually put down in Newcastle and I would have to run through the customs long room to declare the paintings, before rushing on to our connecting flight to Glasgow. As soon as we got home I would quickly clean the frames and lightly go over the paintings before packing them into the van and heading off to see customers I thought would be interested. If I could do a deal quickly enough I could get a cheque off to the auctioneers in time to meet their deadline for payment.

The Christie's people were always so pleasant about everything and always allowed us a month's credit. At one sale I bought paintings worth £40,000 without handing over a penny. I managed to pay them half of the sum at the end of the month and the rest not too much later. They were real gentlemen about it. Sotheby's staff always seemed a rougher lot and on a couple of occasions, when I was late with some payments, wrote to tell me never to set foot in their salerooms again. I didn't take any notice and kept going to the viewings. I guess I was a bit of a chancer in their eyes. On one occasion, when I went to collect my purchases, their credit controller started raging at me, something that I could never imagine happening at Christie's over the odd £10,000.

There was one outstandingly pretty oil painting that I had sold to a wealthy customer, featuring two little girls, one holding a rabbit. When the customer tired of it and asked me to sell it for him, I took it to Christie's in their St James's showroom, where someone in the office said it should be sold in their second-rate saleroom in South Kensington. I doubted if it would fetch more than four or five thousand pounds there and I was certain it deserved better, so I insisted that it was sold at their St James's auction room, where it went for £15,000 to a gentleman who received a grateful kiss from his companion for buying it.

We often used to take Christopher with us when we went to Amsterdam and, when I became too absorbed in walking round and round the auction rooms looking for bargains, he and Grace would slope off for coffee and cake in the cafés.

I enjoyed the London trips to Sotheby's Bond Street auction rooms as well, sometimes going with one of the boys or Grace, having a Guinness and ploughman's lunch at a nearby pub first, followed by chocolates from the luxurious little Charbonnel and Walker shop down the road before making the arrangements to get my purchases back to Scotland.

I relied a lot on Grace's good taste when it came to choosing what to buy. There was a great thrill in seeing a painting that we thought would suit the tastes of a particular customer and then taking the gamble on buying it. Usually we were right, but sometimes we were wrong and the customer said no, or simply couldn't afford the price.

While visiting one of my clients in Ayrshire one day, he told me he had something to show me and led me down to the housemaid's cupboard, where a number of paintings had been stored. One was a portrait of a man called Bateman signed by a painter called Allan Ramsay in 1756. The portrait was painted in Rome when Mr Bateman was conducting the grand tour which all well-bred people did in those days. My client asked me to do some research into it. I discovered that the director of the National Gallery in London considered Ramsay to be a better painter than either Reynolds or Gainsborough, and Timothy Clifford at the National Gallery in Edinburgh offered me £60,000 for it. Sotheby's and Christie's said it would fetch between £60,000 and £80,000 at auction. A well-known dealer in London offered me £12,000 for it and would probably have put it into the gallery with a price tag of anything up to £200,000. It ended up at the National Gallery in Edinburgh, hanging close to a Rembrandt.

In a way, I became a victim of my own success. When things became exciting I was tempted to stretch myself financially, and I was then under pressure to sell enough products to keep the bank happy as well as keeping us and the business going. It's a common problem for small businesses, but I would be the first to admit that business administration is not my strong point. I was good at sniffing out opportunities and I was good at the selling, but my other business skills left something to be desired.

The business might not have been very soundly based financially, but we were certainly enjoying ourselves, going to art auctions, travelling abroad on buying expeditions. There were times, however, when I just wouldn't be able to make any sales and there wouldn't be any money coming into the house. In the past Grace had always been very good about it. When I told her that money was going to be tight for a bit she just went and got herself a job as a sister at a local hospital, working once more with the elderly. The children were bigger by that stage, and we had decided that they were quite capable of looking after themselves for part of the day while Grace was out at work.

We had no idea, of course, of the demons that were building up inside Christopher's head in those years.

In 1985 the world heard about a salvage operation going on in the South China Sea. A Dutch export vessel, the *Geldermelsen*, had sunk after striking a coral reef in 1752. It had been carrying gold and enormous quantities of eighteenth-century Ch'ing Dynasty porcelain, and was being salvaged by a man called Michael Hatcher and his crew. The many thousands of pieces were going to be sold at an auction held by Christie's in the Hilton Hotel, Amsterdam. They called it, with some justification, 'The Sale of the Century', and Grace and I went over to Holland to have a look. The publicity had been worldwide and the hotel ballroom was packed with people wanting to look at – and buy – this extraordinary piece of history.

I was pretty sure that this was the sort of thing that I could sell to my customers. Their walls might be full of paintings, but that didn't mean that they couldn't fit some porcelain and ornaments on to their shelves and surfaces. We found ourselves sitting behind Michael Hatcher, the salvage expert.

I fancied some blue and white export porcelain – produced by the Chinese during the eighteenth century specifically for export to Europe to satisfy the new tea-drinking fashion – including a large fish plate, but the pieces I had my eye on went for many times their estimated prices. On the advice of a dealer sitting next to me, I bought a thousand pieces of tea bowls and saucers at £34 per set and came back to England to set up an exhibition, which attracted large crowds. I ended up making a profit of about £20,000 on the project, which was a lot for me.

All the family was involved in the setting up of the exhibition, which made it an especially happy time for me. Some years later my brother Reg said that it was at that exhibition that he first noticed something strange about the way Grace was behaving. It may be that he was just speaking with the benefit of hindsight, or maybe, even then, unknown to either Grace or me, the illness was beginning to take its hold on her mind, the cells of her brain starting to be destroyed by Alzheimer's. Reg said that she seemed to have lost a little of her sparkle and appeared distracted. At that moment we had too many other things to worry about to be paying close attention to our own health, but soon we would be unable to avoid the truth.

Feeling quite flushed by success, and actually having some money in the bank for a change, I decided we should go out to China to see if we could find more of the same sort of thing to bring back and sell while the demand was still there. It was a good excuse for me to get back to travelling, visiting places I'd never been. The trip was wonderful, and I bought lots of jade and cloisonné (copper and enamel pieces which have been fired and sealed) in Shanghai and Beijing, often buying through the hotels which seemed to have scooped up most of the good pieces from the factories. I was bringing back stuff that people couldn't normally buy in England and taking it round in the van with the pictures, giving myself some more cash flow and helping to disguise the fact that fundamentally the business wasn't making enough profit to support us.

China wasn't the only place to which we travelled. We also went to Eastern Europe, going through Checkpoint Charlie in Berlin to catch the night train to a snow-sprinkled Prague before going on to work at the Leipzig Fair to buy Meissen porcelain. I was never happier than when it was just the two of us in some new and exotic place, learning new things and seeing great sights. It was just like it had been when we had first met and travelled around London, thrilled to be out in the world together. As long as I was with Grace I was completely happy and fulfilled. I couldn't imagine that there was a luckier man on earth.

CHAPTER FIVE

A First Mind is Overthrown

Children aren't happy with nothing to ignore,
And that is what parents were created for.

OGDEN NASH

G race and I had our differences from time to time, like any
couple. It would have been very strange if we had not.
There was a period when I became interested in religion,
tempted by my brother to attend a few Jehovah's Witnesses'
meetings and becoming quite enthusiastic about their ideas,
as many new converts to any religion tend to be.

Grace was very much opposed to traditional western
religions, being much more interested in the esoteric
philosophical ideas of the East. They suited her quiet,
thoughtful, accepting view of life. She behaved in a good
Christian way but preferred to go to classes for meditation and
other eastern spiritual techniques than to attend meetings or
go to church to worship. She was not evangelical about her
beliefs, not wanting to convert anyone who wasn't already

seeking something, but she was equally unwilling to be preached to by people who believed they knew better than her. When I am enthusiastic about something I tend to become very evangelical – it must be the salesman in me – and sometimes we would argue as a result, but we would always make up quickly. Neither of us could bear to be cross with the other for long and, because Grace was so placid and accepting about most things, when she did stick up for herself I knew she really meant what she was saying and that I would be unlikely to be able to change her opinion.

Although we had moved east out of Glasgow for a while, it was hard to sell art around the Edinburgh area because of all the established galleries. So we went back to Glasgow and bought a beautiful semi-detached house which had once been owned by a timber merchant and was full of the most beautiful tropical woods. It cost me £8,000, which seemed an awful lot at the time, but it was worth it to live in such pleasant surroundings.

It was a time of change. I know that in some circles the subject of sex was being discussed a great deal at that time, but, like the vast majority of men, I didn't get to read the articles in *Cosmopolitan* or the writings of Germaine Greer. I continued to behave as most men had behaved for centuries. Grace, on the other hand, was a thoroughly modern woman, and was generous to me in bed. If I was selfish about my ways, she was too shy and polite a person to protest about such things to my face. She did once lay a book of alternative sexual positions on my desk, where I was bound to find it. She never said anything about it, and to my eternal shame I never asked her why she had done that or what I could do to please her more, until eventually it was too late for her to be able to give me an answer.

I understand now that, as the years go by, it is all too easy to get into familiar habits and for the process to become mechanical. Sex should be like travel: you should always be moving on to new experiences and new sights, learning new things about yourself and your partner, not returning to the same, safe, comfortable destination every year.

That book lying on my desk should have been a wake-up call. As it was I flicked through it with curiosity, much as I might have flicked through an art book, and then put it away in a drawer somewhere, not wanting the boys to come across it. If I did make any effort to change my ways it was minimal and short-lived, and Grace must have resigned herself to the fact that things were not likely to improve. She never raised the subject again.

There must have been many other petty irritations involved in living with me, and maybe some that were not so petty. I often, for instance, used to hang the pictures I had bought around the house, so that we could enjoy them until I sold them or had room for them in the van. Grace would just have got used to them when I would arbitrarily decide to take them off on the road with me, leaving her with an empty wall and never consulting her. It must have been very frustrating for someone trying to build a nice home for herself and her family.

On another occasion she had an azalea bush of which she was particularly fond; one day a lady artist came to call, took a liking to the bush and cut off the best bit, saying she would paint it. She did, indeed, produce a good painting, which I then hung in the house. But as soon as a neighbour made me an offer I sold it, leaving Grace with a mutilated bush and no painting. I wish now I had been more considerate at such times and consulted her more often about her thoughts and feelings, because it wasn't long before she wouldn't be able to understand her own feelings any more, let alone articulate them. I could have made life better for her in so many ways, if I had just thought about it more instead of doing the first thing that came into my head all the time.

Grace was not a great one for making friends, seeming to be quite happy with her family, and with the colleagues and patients she encountered when she was working. There was one woman, however, with whom she got on particularly well. Maggie Brown was a speech therapist who lived across the road with her schoolteacher husband, Allan. Maggie was a pleasant, rotund woman and when she came to visit our house Grace would stock up on thick cream and chocolate cakes. They would sometimes chat for hours, well into the night. Grace was wonderful at listening to other people's problems. (For many years she worked for the Samaritans, answering their phones and helping with the assessment of new volunteers. She and another lady used to organise visits and dances to allow introverted callers to socialise.) I'm ashamed to say that I sometimes became rather put out at being left on my own upstairs and used to go down after midnight and say that I wanted Grace in bed. She would be quite upset, and rightly so, when I behaved like that.

The Browns had very different views to us on many things, particularly medicine. They were great believers in the power of doctors and hated anything that could be described as alternative medicine. When I pointed out to them in the course of a heated discussion that 40,000 people die every year due to the adverse effects of prescribed drugs, and many hundreds of thousands more are maimed, some permanently, they said they thought it was a price worth paying for the many who do survive. I had very different views, which I suspect Grace would sometimes have liked me to keep to myself in company.

But beneath these normal surface irritations, which I guess you would find in most long-lasting marriages, there was a far worse crisis brewing that neither of us had any idea was on the way.

Christopher, our youngest son, was developing an illness that would make his and our lives almost impossible in the coming years. It was like having a giant killer shark lurking invisibly beneath the calm waters of some sunny beach resort, as we continued with our own lives above the water, splashing happily about, oblivious to the dangers that were approaching from the dark, mysterious depths below us.

We knew that Christopher was different, but that didn't cause me any worries. I myself had always been attracted to different paths through life, and liked people who saw things from a new angle. I think that was why I enjoyed the company of artists as much as I did. But there was something more to Christopher than just being different, something far more dark and dangerous.

Whereas Anne, Clifford and Kenneth had worked hard at school, with Anne going on to teacher training college and qualifying as a teacher, Clifford going to Glasgow University and gaining a science degree, and Kenneth starting his own computer design company, Christopher never really studied anything. He never passed any exams or achieved anything. As I had never achieved anything either at school, this didn't seem too much of a problem to me. Perhaps I should have seen the shark's fin appearing in the waves when I read those early school reports, but I was too busy having fun in the shallows and told Grace I was sure he would find something that interested him in time.

As time went on, we seemed to be unable to talk to him rationally. If we tried to strike up a conversation about how he was feeling he started to tell us that he believed people were after him. He thought we should do something about helping him stop his oppressors, but he could never be clear who they were or why they were after him. He just knew they were there. Since he seldom ventured out of the house and invited no friends in to visit, we couldn't imagine who these people might be, beyond shadows in his brain. He believed the security services were after him. He was so convincing in his arguments that to begin with I thought there might be some truth in what he was saying; why would you doubt the word of your own child when you know nothing about what is going on in their life and their head?

I actually went to talk to a lawyer about helping him with his persecutors. But even as I told the lawyer what it was that was worrying Christopher, I could hear the madness of my own words. It might sound convincing when he was actually telling us what was going on in his head, but as soon as I tried to convey his worries to a third party I could see the transparent paranoia of them and felt foolish for ever having been swept up in such delusions.

At the time, Christopher had been practising knife-throwing at a large piece of plywood in the back garden. Grace and I thought nothing of it, and the first we knew of the impending disaster was when he was seventeen years old and the police brought him home one day, telling us that they'd picked him up at a railway station with six or seven butcher's knives on him. It seemed he had armed himself against an imagined enemy. Had the weapons merely been hidden about his person no one would have been any the wiser, but he had been playing with them in full view of alarmed passers-by, as if wanting everyone to be aware that he was armed and dangerous in case they were considering attacking him.

We were shocked. We knew enough about mental illness to understand what this sort of behaviour indicated. Our youngest son, who as a small boy had looked so like his fair, delicately boned mother, had grown up to be a schizophrenic while I had been looking the other way. The shark had surfaced amongst us with a terrifying speed and there was no chance we could ever go back to the way things had been before. It looked as if he might even have to go to prison for the knife incident. We could only imagine what sort of effect such an experience would have on his already unhinged mind.

It may take me a while to notice that something is wrong, but once I have recognised a problem I have never been one to try to cover it up. I saw nothing to be ashamed or secretive about in Christopher's plight – quite the opposite. I wanted to talk about this new nightmare as much as possible in the hope that I would manage to find some way to straighten out my thoughts on the subject, or that someone else might come up with some suggestions as to what we could do. When I mentioned the problem to one of my customers, who was a lawyer, he told me of another young lawyer he had seen perform in a case like this. I immediately made contact, desperate to do anything I could to stop Christopher being treated as a criminal, and he agreed to do what he could. 'Perform' is the right word for the way this man pleaded in court, and he managed to convince them that Christopher needed help not punishment.

In order to help him we needed first to try to find out what was wrong. We needed to know our enemy before we could fight him. Both Grace and I had experience of dealing with the mental problems of old age but dealing with a disturbed young man was something new to us. Specialists told us that our son had a sort of dementia that tended to attack younger brains. They put him on heavy anti-psychotic medication and he started going in and out of hospital for various treatments.

The shadowy world of mental illness is still a baffling one to the majority of the medical profession. At times Christopher was committed to some terrible wards filled with deeply troubled souls and understaffed by harassed nurses and doctors. As the years went by we had him at home most of the time, but the demons were becoming stronger. Every time he made a suicide attempt, taking pills or slashing at his wrists with razor blades, he would have to be taken back into hospital to be stabilised again with drugs.

I felt he needed something to do in order to connect better with the real world, and tried to involve him in the business, taking him with me on trips and getting him to do some of the framing of the pictures, which he was good at. But it didn't seem to help his state of mind. He became involved with the National Front and their very right wing crusade; perhaps it was a reaction to me and Grace and our left-wing history. Christopher started to pin up pictures of Hitler in his room and distribute leaflets around the area. His brothers had both met and been influenced by National Front people at some stage, but it seemed to have been more of a passing phase with them.

It all made me feel very uncomfortable, but then I rationalised it away, telling myself that no doubt my youthful communist leanings must have seemed just as alarming to my Conservative parents. We can all hope that our children will share our visions of how the world should be, but we can't force them to.

Eventually, Christopher was the only one of the children

left at home. Anne had become a teacher and married a lawyer, Clifford had gone to university and Kenneth had started making his way in the business world. Christopher was left in his bedroom or the television room on his own, not wanting to have to talk to Grace or me more than he had to, alone in his frightening private world while his brothers and sister got on with their lives. He seemed to have lost all patience with us, and we didn't know how to bridge the communication gap that was opening up between us and growing wider every day.

One day we heard noises coming from the television room and when we went to see what was happening we discovered Christopher hurling things around in what seemed to be an uncontrollable fury. Windows and picture frames were shattering, sending glass splintering in all directions. Cutlery, glasses and the television joined the rest of the room's contents on the floor as he ranted and raved. It wasn't the first time he'd run amok like this but it was certainly the most ferocious explosion of violence. There was nothing I could do to control him. I had no option but to call the police and ask for help.

Initially Grace and I took shelter in the garage, although there was hardly any room amidst the clutter; then some neighbours, a surgeon and his wife, offered us sanctuary in their house. When the police arrived, fully equipped with riot shields, they took Christopher back to hospital to be stabilised once more with drugs. Imagine the feelings of a father who has to call the police to help him control his son in his own home.

We became members of the National Schizophrenia Fellowship, and there was always information on the latest ideas and theories arriving through the post, which Grace and I would read avidly, searching for clues about our youngest son's condition. One day there was a report about a nutritionist named Anne Good who produced a newspaper called *FIND* (Food Intolerance and Nutritional Deficiency). Anne was a State Registered Nurse and was married to a psychiatrist. She had spent her life nursing, much of the time in Africa. I had always believed strongly in the power of nutrition to affect both our physical and mental health, and I felt sure it was a path we should explore. The traditional medical establishment was still very doubtful about such things: certainly it accepted the values of proteins, carbohydrates, fats and vitamins in a normal diet, but it was not ready for the suggestion that mental illness could result from biochemical imbalances in the brain, which could be corrected by dietary means.

We contacted Anne Good and explained our problem. She recommended we take Christopher to Nutrition Associates in York to be assessed for allergies and intolerances. This seemed to us like a much more positive way forward. Until that point we had just been trying to force him to take medication that he didn't want to take in order to subdue him, rather than trying to tackle the causes of the problem. He was now a fully grown man in his twenties and there were limits to what we could make him do against his will. If we could find some answers in his diet, we thought it would be relatively easy to convince him to change his eating habits and take supplements.

Grace took him along to York and, after undergoing tests, he was given a prescription for vitamin and mineral supplements that they believed would help to redress the imbalances in his system. It was a steep learning curve for both of us. We discovered, for instance, that without sufficient quantities of zinc people can suffer irritability, insomnia and paranoia, becoming unduly suspicious of others. Four per cent of those labelled schizophrenic, we read, are simply allergic to the gluten in wheat and can be cured with a gluten-free diet. Tests done on schizophrenic patients in America showed that those who were on milk- and cereal-free diets were ready to be discharged from hospital twice as fast as those on control diets, but when wheat-gluten was added to the cereal-free diet the advantage was eradicated. Another study of fifty-three patients showed that ninety-two per cent of them were allergic to at least one or more common substances such as wheat, corn, cow's milk, tobacco and petrochemical hydrocarbons.

It seemed unarguable that many types of schizophrenia would respond to suitable diet supplementation, and that giving sufferers the right vitamins and minerals would cost just a few pence a day, as opposed to the thousands of pounds a year it could cost to provide custodial care. In another test on a hundred patients admitted to a psychiatric hospital, eighty per cent were found to have a physical illness that hadn't been diagnosed before. In over half of them the physical illness was thought to have caused or contributed to the psychiatric symptoms and sixty-one per cent of them were cured of their psychiatric symptoms the moment the underlying physical disorders were treated. It seemed likely, from what we read, that a large proportion of the patients in psychiatric wards were not actually mentally ill, but were suffering from physical illnesses which displayed mental symptoms.

Allergies affect all of us to some degree, even the most mentally well balanced. They can have any number of different effects on us. If it is an outward sign like a rash or a shortness of breath it is obvious, but changes in mood and behaviour can be harder to quantify. An allergy can make us irritable, restless or overactive, or it can have the opposite effect and make us feel tired and lethargic. It can create mental confusion, slowness of thought, depression and impaired memory.

Very often people suffer from these symptoms all their lives without ever knowing why or what to do about them. Usually they have reached this condition after many years of suffering other physical and mental problems. They often have thick medical files, filled with many reports of mysterious complaints that can be traced back to allergic reactions within the brain. I am convinced that in almost all cases of mental disease, the problems stem from food and chemical allergies. Instead of prescribing mood-altering drugs, electric-shock therapy and psychotherapy, all of which generally lead the patient further downhill in the long term, doctors need to be addressing what is causing the allergy in the first place, so that it can be removed from the sufferer's diet. (For the record, I believe that psychotherapy can help in the short term, but the practice, in Britain at least, is still in a drug rut.)

The more we read and researched, the more sure we became that this was the path down which we should be leading Christopher. We were certain that if we could get his diet and supplements right we could release him from his demons and he would be able to get on with living and enjoying his adult life.

We followed the nutritionist's instructions to the letter and immediately saw a dramatic improvement in Christopher's levels of behaviour. He started to go out swimming and exercising, and responded well when I suggested we go to different events together. Unfortunately he was also seeing a psychiatrist who, like so many medical practitioners in those days, didn't believe that vitamins and supplements made any difference, and it didn't take much effort for him to persuade Christopher to stop bothering to take them with a few dismissive and mocking phrases. Christopher certainly wasn't going to believe the theories of his eccentric parents over the words of a psychiatrist who had all the trappings of a professional establishment behind him.

Throughout the early years of Christopher's illness, of course, I was out in the van earning a living for much of the time, and Grace was left at home to take all the strain. Although I always missed Grace desperately, I have to admit that I would also experience a feeling of selfish relief as I drove away in the uncomplicated company of Shandy, the randy mongrel, leaving behind the oppressive, troubled atmosphere that enveloped the house when Christopher was there. Grace had far fewer chances of respite, and for a mother to have to see her child in such distress must have been unimaginably hard. To find your son with his wrists slashed or his stomach filled with paracetamol must take a terrible toll on your own state of mind.

In one of his later attempts to overdose, he even fed tablets to the dog, (by that time Shandy had passed on and been replaced by a handsome Irish Water Spaniel called Meissen). Both Christopher and the dog were saved by stomach pumping, although Meissen was never fully himself again and died prematurely a while later. It was impossible to predict when these acts of self-destruction would happen. They would seem to us to come out of the blue, so even on the quiet days there was always a feeling that potential disaster was lurking beneath the surface.

I think that, because of our backgrounds in nursing and social work, Grace and I were able to cope for longer than many parents would have been able to do, but that didn't mean that it wasn't a strain. Being a professional nurse is one thing, seeing your own child suffering from dementia on a daily basis is quite another.

I was constantly reading books and articles, trying to find new ideas and possible answers. I came across the work of Dr Carl Pfeiffer, whose clinic in Princeton, New Jersey, Grace and I would visit later when we became aware that she had Alzheimer's. He had summed up well what appeared to have happened to Christopher, explaining that the thing schizophrenics all have in common is extreme misery, not enjoying their lives and feeling that they are in prison. He explained that they don't feel free to make proper choices for themselves, many becoming suicidal and many being unable to perform even simple tasks or get themselves jobs. Some of them hear voices; others see floors rolling away in front of them or become paranoid. Our understanding of the condition was growing all the time but we still had no idea how to cope with it.

Although my business was still fundamentally going downhill, I seemed to have got on top of the cash-flow problems that had been dogging us, and Grace was able to give up working once more. That meant she was at home with Christopher nearly all the time, unless he was having a spell in hospital. But, while the grasp of the demons on our son's brain continued to ebb and flow, the disease that was eating away at Grace's own brain must also have been establishing its corrosive hold all that time, and I still knew nothing about it.

CHAPTER 6

THE DISEASE INTRODUCES ITSELF

Only reason can convince us of those three
fundamental truths without recognition of which there
can be no effective liberty: that what we believe is
not necessarily true; that what we like is not necessarily
good: and that all questions are open.

CLIVE BELL

One evening Grace and I were sitting next to one another in the kitchen, and she was organising herself to do some sewing while we sipped our cocoa and chatted, winding down from the day and preparing ourselves for bed. I loved those moments together; they were the pictures I held in my mind whenever I was away on my own in the van.

Grace was having trouble threading the needle that she was going to use to reattach a fallen button. Everyone has difficulty threading needles, particularly once their eyes begin to descend into middle age and the details of the distance become sharper than the things which are under our noses, but this appeared to be something more.

She didn't seem to be able to co-ordinate the necessary

motor skills needed to line the tip of the thread with the needle's eye; she couldn't instruct her fingers to make the precise movement needed to guide it through that sliver of steel. For a second I thought perhaps she was dropping a hint that I should sew on my own button – she was not above reminding me that there had been a women's liberation movement which had largely passed me by – but I soon dismissed this idea because she seemed to be concerned by what was happening between her eyes and the tips of her fingers. Very few things ruffled Grace's calm, but I could see she was distressed.

'Maybe you need to get your eyes checked,' I suggested.

'I don't think it's my eyes,' she replied. 'I can see quite clearly. I just don't seem to be able to make my fingers do as they're told.'

'It's probably nothing,' I assured her and at that stage I didn't think it was.

Once you have been alerted to the presence of something new and strange in your life, you sometimes realise it has been there for a while and that you have been ignoring it, perhaps from choice or convenience, or simply because your thoughts were elsewhere. When people discover that their partner has been unfaithful, for instance, they often look back over the preceding months and realise that all the clues of the betrayal were there, if they had just chosen to translate them into suspicions.

Grace had suffered a few small lapses of memory recently, but nothing that you couldn't put down to someone in their mid-fifties with other things preoccupying their mind. It is sometimes hard to focus on the day-to-day business of living when you have bigger problems pressing on you all the time, and as you grow older you sometimes fail to remember things that might seem unimportant.

Once I'd realised something was wrong I started to notice other things. Grace's appearance was no longer as immaculate as it had once been and she would often forget to brush her hair or even to put on appropriate clothes to go out. More than once I found her wearing odd shoes or putting a jumper on back to front.

Things began to appear in odd places, like an address book and diary in the fridge or a plastic container filled with butter melting in the oven. She would forget to lock doors, or would lose keys which had always been kept in the same place. Her handbag would turn up in the most unlikely hiding places and she would swear that she had no memory of putting it there. In conversation she started to repeat the same questions, completely forgetting that I had already answered them, and would have no memory of something which had happened just a few minutes before. She would phone a friend to ask a question, and then do exactly the same thing again an hour or two later.

'I'm so stupid,' Grace would grumble when she caught herself making these mistakes.

'You're not stupid, Grace,' I assured her. 'You have never been stupid in your life.'

'But I get so confused, about everything, and then I do things which I can't explain.'

'We're all getting older,' I said. 'These things happen.' But I knew in my heart that this was now more than the normal forgetfulness of advancing years.

Gradually, we were alerted to danger. We realised that the lapses in memory had been more than the usual carelessness of the middle-aged mind. We had both done geriatric nursing, had watched as dementia took hold of previously agile minds and gradually removed all their skills and abilities. We both knew that what we had spotted in Grace could be the very first signs of Alzheimer's.

I don't remember feeling particularly panicked at that stage, just determined to combat its onset in every way possible, slow down its monstrous approach for as long as I could and look after Grace to the very best of my ability for as long as we were both alive. Some things in life are inevitable, and you simply have to accept and deal with them as they occur. Alzheimer's is one of those things. Grace accepted the possibility of the disease as calmly as she accepted everything else that life threw at her.

'I think we need to start thinking about the future,' she said one day, 'how we'll cope if I get worse.'

'You don't have to worry,' I assured her. 'We'll always cope, whatever happens.'

I had by that stage heard of the Princetown Brain Bio Center in New Jersey, having studied nutritional therapy when trying to get a handle on Christopher's problems. It seemed, from everything I had read or heard about it, to be the best place in the world to go to for the sort of treatment that we both believed in so strongly. We didn't bother to go to our own local doctor because we didn't think he would be able to tell us anything we didn't know from our own experiences; we feared he would just have tried to talk us into using drugs that neither of us believed in, trying to suppress the symptoms as they had done with Christopher, rather than looking for ways to prepare Grace's body to be as healthy as possible in order to fight the illness in every way it could. Inevitably we would lose the war, because we are all mortal, but there were going to be a good few battles along the way that we very well might win if we laid our plans carefully enough.

I have always been doubtful as to whether traditional doctors are always the best people to go to for help. I am a great fan of the monthly magazine *What Doctors Don't Tell You*, which is written for the lay person and exposes many of the dangers of modern medicine, providing good, safe, efficient alternatives. I believe the magazine has saved thousands of lives.

The Brain Bio Center was founded by Dr Carl Pfeiffer, a psychiatrist with degrees in medicine, chemistry and pharmacology. Pfeiffer himself had recently passed away, but he had laid the necessary foundations and his methods were still being practised at the clinic, which seemed to enjoy a tremendous success rate. Whereas most psychiatrists believe in treating mental illnesses with drugs, Dr Pfeiffer believed the problems nearly always stemmed from biochemical imbalances in the body. Every single one of his treatments was dietary, with the primary aim of getting the patients off their drug crutches, restoring the biochemical balance within their systems that nature intended so that they were in the very best of health.

'There are a hundred ways to go crazy,' he once wrote, 'and I believe every one of them has a biochemical cause.' Such imbalances, he believed, could be corrected with diet, using combinations of vitamins and minerals. He was convinced that by using drugs you were merely turning patients into manageable zombies, rather than attempting to return them to a natural state of good mental health. Anyone treated by him, he claimed, could lead a perfectly full life in the outside world. That was a message we were very open to receiving.

He himself had practised orthodox medicine until the age of fifty-one, when he suffered a heart attack which made him take some time off and look objectively at what he was doing with his life and what he truly believed in. The insights he gained during that sabbatical persuaded him to set up his own clinic and treat patients his own way. The message he was conveying came as a welcome relief to many people like us who had been thinking along the same lines but lacked the scientific skills to put their theories into practice. His success rate with patients was staggering, and it wasn't long before the clinic was seeing 5,000 people a year and gaining a reputation worldwide.

Other psychiatrists continued to dismiss him as a crank for some years, but his extremely high success rate eventually forced all but the most stubborn of them to start taking him seriously and to admit that there had to be some foundation to his claims. With his methods he was able to cure epileptics, manic depressives and schizophrenics, enabling them to come off their drug therapy. There were case studies published that told of patients who hadn't spoken for years suddenly finding their voice again once treated by him, becoming as talkative as they were before their illnesses struck.

He also believed that the work he was doing with individuals had wider implications for society as a whole. He was sure there was a close connection between violent crime and the effects of severe mineral imbalances in the brain of the perpetrator. A man who had killed more than twenty people in San Diego, for instance, was found to have the highest hair cadmium content ever recorded. Cadmium is a toxic anti-nutrient found in cigarettes. In recent years it has become generally accepted that almost 100 per cent of the world's criminal prison population has some sort of chemical imbalance in their system, which makes them behave the way they do. Imagine the effect on the world if all these people could be treated from childhood to make them more balanced human beings, simply by changing their diet and giving them supplements.

I was convinced that the staff at Pfeiffer's centre would be the best people to help Grace, and I wrote them an enquiry letter. Almost by return of post they sent us a lengthy psychological questionnaire, asking all the sorts of questions that we would have to have answered in a consultation, so it was useful to get them out of the way before we arrived. Visiting such a place was obviously going to be an expensive business anyway as it was in America, and anything we could do to keep our time there to a minimum was good. We sent the form back with our deposit and were given an appointment. We flew over to New York and booked ourselves into a hotel not far from the clinic.

Both of us were coping with things as they happened, trying not to worry about anything until it actually happened and concentrating all our energies on making Grace's system as healthy and balanced as possible on a day-to-day basis, so it could put up the best possible fight against the approaching enemy. Our experiences as professional nurses and with Christopher made us completely realistic about the sort of things that can go wrong with brains and, while that meant that we probably had a clearer idea of what sort of horrors we would be confronting in the future, we also knew that they were survivable. We had both lived amongst dementia sufferers and knew what it was going to be like. We were just taking each day as it came, determined to do whatever we could to defer the inevitable, while continuing to enjoy ourselves, and one another, as much as we always had.

At the clinic Grace was seen by one of the doctors, who had his wife present at all times. The whole process took several hours as he undertook some tests and eventually confirmed what we already knew, that Grace had Alzheimer's. That was our first official diagnosis, and we never bothered to ask anyone else for a second opinion because we both knew, in our hearts, that it was correct. He then gave us a list of the supplements that he believed, from looking at the test results, Grace's system needed, many of which they had in stock at the clinic so we could purchase them then and there.

Although we thought we might be able to slow down the disease's progress, and lessen some of the worst symptoms, we already knew we had left it too late to actually avoid it. Perhaps, had Grace been taking those supplements all her adult life, the disease would never have been able to get a foothold. Or perhaps it wouldn't have managed to break through for another ten or twenty years. Personally, I believe strongly that if people are diagnosed early in their lives by nutritionists, and then stick to the diets and supplements that are recommended, they could end up substantially increasing their life expectancy, and greatly improving the standard of their well-being during those years. Myself, I would like to think I'm going to make it to 110 without any trouble, substantially cutting down my chances of being struck down by many of the common killers like heart disease. But it may be that I also came too late to the right diet, and that something unnatural was already at work in my body before I started to pay attention to everything I ate and did.

By the end of the afternoon at the clinic we felt almost relieved. Our worst fears might have been confirmed, but at least we felt now that we were doing something positive and we knew who the enemy was for sure. When we got back home, our luggage filled with tablets, Grace started making phone calls. She rang round our relatives to inform them that she had been diagnosed with Alzheimer's. Her voice was completely steady and matter-of-fact as she conveyed information that was shocking news to them but not to us. She showed no signs of fear of what now lay ahead, and I don't remember either of us ever shedding a tear or voicing any regrets about the past or disappointment about the future. We only looked forward, putting all our energies into making plans and preparing for the battle.

For a while we continued with our lives, me out on the road trying to sell the art, Grace at home with Christopher, when he wasn't in hospital. She would suffer occasional lapses of memory, and I could see now that some of her old sparkle was beginning to desert her, her eyes taking on a slightly vacant look some of the time; but she was still able to look after herself for a few days at a time. All the time I was away, however, I was thinking about her, trying to work out what was the best thing to do. I knew it would not be long before I would need to be at home all the time, but how would I make a living?

The business was not doing well, and I knew that I wouldn't be able to sell it for any sort of profit. In fact I might have to get rid of it quickly just to meet my debt to the bank. I was reluctant to make that move, having enjoyed the life so much and knowing that once I'd given it up it was very unlikely I would ever get back to it. The stress of trying to decide what direction to go in next was getting to me, splitting me between my worries about leaving Grace and about not being able to earn enough money to support us both at home.

I knew it would not be long before some major life decisions would need to be taken, but waiting for the solution to come was an agonising business. I'm good at being spontaneous, and brave when it comes to taking risks, but I am terrible when faced with logical choices and important decisions which have to be made.

Alzheimer's is progressive and degenerative, attacking the brain and causing memory loss in the early stages. It then moves relentlessly forward, wearing away the sufferer's intellectual ability until eventually they're unable to control their thoughts or their bodies in any way. To begin with they lose the ability to do small everyday tasks like running a bath, cooking a meal or going to the toilet. Ordinary life begins to become unmanageable and they have to have someone with them at all times to take over the tasks they can no longer remember how to do for themselves.

In many cases this stage is accompanied with changes of mood, behaviour and personality. The sufferers can become challenging and aggressive, like small uncontrollable children throwing tantrums, even when such behaviour is completely out of character for them. The terrible difference is that they aren't small children who can be picked up and held tightly until they calm down. They are fully grown adults, and so their behaviour seems all the more threatening and frightening to those who witness it. They can actually land punches that do some damage to anyone unlucky enough to be in their path.

Whereas with children there are things you can do and say which will teach them that such behaviour is unacceptable and that they must adapt it, the Alzheimer's sufferer has no such ability to learn, no such power to develop or improve. Things will only ever get worse with time, and that can make the carer's task seem far more onerous than the task faced by the parent of an angry child. It is when faced with that sort of behaviour that so many people decide it is time to sedate the patient in order to make them manageable, leaving them sitting staring ahead of them like a vegetable, or dozing in bed.

Alzheimer's is a primary form of dementia, but different forms of dementia stem from the same diseases of the nervous system, and many people suffer from more than one type. It is a disease that is particularly prevalent in the developed world, where about one-and-a-half per cent of sixty-five-year-olds suffer from it. That percentage doubles every four years, so that thirty per cent of eighty-year-olds are afflicted.

That is such a shocking statistic that I probably need to state it again. If anyone you know, whether it is either of your parents, your partner or a close relative, lives to be eighty there is almost a one-in-three chance that they will fall prey to Alzheimer's. With ever-increasing life expectancy in the West, nearly all of us will have at least three people close to us who will reach that age, which means that virtually all of us will be touched by this illness at some stage of our lives. It may be, of course, that it will be us who are the sufferers and our partners who are the carers. So everyone reading this book is very likely to have to face this problem at some stage in his or her later years, either as a sufferer or a carer.

In the developing world, however, dementia of any type is rare. Our predisposition towards Alzheimer's may be partly caused by the fact that we live longer since it is, generally speaking, an illness of the old. But it may also be to do with the diets we eat, filled as they are with processed foods, chemicals and additives. Or it may be that in the developing world, where families tend to live more communally, sufferers are not reported to the authorities, but are simply looked after and loved by other family members who would no more call themselves 'carers' than a mother would describe herself as a carer for her baby.

Most of us would like to continue extending our natural lifespans, so that is always going to remain a contributing factor. It is the dietary side of the equation, therefore, that we can address most easily and to the greatest effect. To start with, an intake of antioxidants, particularly vitamins C and E, may lower the risk of us developing Alzheimer's. Dutch researchers collected data on 5,395 subjects who were at least fifty-five years old and free of dementia. After an average of six years, 197 of these people had dementia, of whom 146 were diagnosed as suffering from Alzheimer's. After adjusting the figures to take account of risk factors such as age, sex, overall mental health, alcohol intake, education (poor education is associated with having a less active mind), smoking and diet, the researchers concluded that a high dietary intake of vitamins C and E was associated with a nearly twenty per cent reduced risk of Alzheimer's.

Researchers at the Rush Institute for Healthy Ageing in Chicago found that the more foods containing vitamin E a person consumed, the lower their risk of developing Alzheimer's. To reach this conclusion, data was collected on 815 community-dwelling men and women aged sixty-five and above, who were without Alzheimer's. Their diets were monitored for nearly four years and those with the highest dietary vitamin E intake had a seventy per cent lower risk of developing Alzheimer's compared to those with the lowest intakes. The researchers' overall conclusion, however, suggested that Alzheimer's is largely an environmental illness.

A recent study, reported in *The Lancet*, referred to research published in *Archives of Neurology*. It stated that investigators from John Hopkins University, Maryland, examined data on 4,740 people aged over 65 years, of which 304 showed signs of Alzheimer's disease. Each of the participants was questioned about their intake of vitamin supplements. Around 17% reported taking vitamin C or E and another 20% used multivitamins, but without a high dose of either E or C. The researchers found that people taking both vitamins were 78% less likely to show signs of Alzheimer's than those not taking the combination. No benefit was found for taking either vitamin in isolation.

Another study, looking at 2,459 healthy, community-dwelling residents in a non-industrial city in Nigeria, compared them with a similar group of healthy, community-dwelling African-Americans living in a busy, industrialised US city. Both groups were followed for around five years and the rates for Alzheimer's and other forms of dementia were more than twice as high in the African-Americans, suggesting that exposure to western pollutants, heavy metals and processed foods may have had a role to play in the development of the diseases.

Vitamin E has a particular antioxidant role on cell membranes, at times working in tandem with vitamin C and interacting with vitamin A, the B-complex vitamins and selenium. It prevents toxic interaction with fats and oxygen in cells and so plays a vital role in maintaining the cell's integrity and use of oxygen. As an immune system enhancer, vitamin E especially protects against lung damage from pollution.

A national study of 1,000 American patients showed that vitamin E supplements reduced the risk of oral cancer by half. As for treatment, of forty-three patients at a cancer centre in Texas who had pre-cancerous oral lesions treated with vitamin E, nearly half improved and a fifth showed evidence of cell improvement after six months.

Selenium, a substance often found in seafood, works in partnership with vitamin E to protect against cancer and to prevent cell membrane damage. This mineral protects against environmental and chemical sensitivities and enhances the body's antibacterial and antiviral defences. A variety of animal and human studies point to its ability to inhibit colon, cervical, breast and liver cancers. A study in

Finland, for instance, found that blood levels of selenium were significantly lower in men who went on to develop stomach cancer.

In all the attention focused on antioxidants, the role of essential fatty acids in protecting and treating cancer and maintaining a healthy immune system is often overlooked. There are two kinds of essential fatty acids – omega-3 and omega-6. They are called 'essential' because the body needs them but cannot manufacture them for itself. No one is sure how essential fatty acids counteract cancer, but it may be to do with their ability to bind to protein and so prevent the toxic action of tumour cells.

Apart from the above, there may be other elements in food that can protect a body against cancer. Researchers from John Hopkins University in Baltimore found that broccoli, Brussels sprouts, cauliflower, cress and other vegetables of the *cruciferae* family all contain a chemical called sulphoraphane, which apparently has anti-cancer properties.

When put down in black and white like that, it all sounds rather complicated and difficult to follow. In reality most carers never need to understand why or how the various different vitamins and supplements work, they simply need wise and professional guidance on what to take and when to take it.

The following two lists made up Grace's daily treatment in the early stages of the disease:

SUPPLEMENTS

2,000µg vitamin B12

500mg niacin

250mg vitamin B6

200µg selenium

1,000 IU vitamin E

1 Solgar VM 75 multivitamin with minerals

800µg folic acid

4,000mg vitamin C with citrus bioflavonoids

1 Solgar advanced carotenoid complex

45mg elemental zinc

no drugs of any kind

GRACE'S DIET

allergy-free foods (no chicken, rice or chocolate in
Grace's case)

mackerel or herring three times a week

plenty of fruit and vegetables

organic food whenever possible

no alcohol

bottled water to avoid the chemicals in tap water

The battle against the disease had commenced. Our main
weapon: as much knowledge as possible.

CHAPTER SEVEN

A New Life

Love is so simple.

JACQUES PRÉVERT

A s things grew gradually more confused inside her head, the need to change our life radically became more urgent in order to achieve the sort of lifestyle that Grace needed if she was to continue functioning as part of normal society. Grace had been diagnosed with Alzheimer's in 1990 at the age of fifty-six. By 1992, it had become clear that she couldn't go on being in the house on her own much longer while I went out to work. The travelling gallery, however much I loved it, was going to have to go.

Closing the business, however, was not going to be a straightforward affair. It was still not going well, carrying far too much debt and not creating enough cash flow. I should have called it a day much earlier, as the market grew harder and the interest payments to the bank kept mounting up, but

I kidded myself that if I just kept all the balls in the air for a bit longer something would turn up which would change everything and I would be able to take some profit before closing down.

The time for kidding myself, though, was over as it became increasingly obvious that no miracle was going to present itself in time to bail me out. I'd filled all my regular customers' houses with art, and they'd spent all they intended, or could afford, to spend. In my desperation to keep going and my refusal to accept when a good thing was over, I was driving around for hours every day, running up terrible petrol bills, and coming home with no sales.

The whole concept had been a child of its moment, and that moment had long since passed. Competition was increasing with new galleries opening up in Glasgow, and I was unable to concentrate on the selling as I grew more and more worried about Grace's ability to look after herself when I was away. I would phone home regularly and she often sounded confused or puzzled to hear from me. Returning from one trip I discovered that she had been living almost exclusively on chocolate bars and milky instant coffee ever since I left, unable to get her mind around preparing any meal at all, let alone one that contained all the vitamins she needed. I became increasingly reluctant to leave her.

As I started to be around the house more I noticed that we were receiving a lot of phone calls where, when I picked up the receiver, the line went dead. I had so many things on my mind I didn't pay too much attention, assuming it was just someone who had been given a wrong number and was too shy to speak to a stranger. Then, one Sunday, when I got home from church, I found a man I had never set eyes on before sitting in the drawing room. Although I didn't recognise him he seemed to know Grace well, and I felt an uncomfortable stab of suspicion mixed with alarm and possibly even a hint of jealousy. How was it possible that the love of my life had an apparently friendly relationship with a man I had never heard of? Grace seemed entirely unperturbed by the situation.

When I enquired who he was, they told me they had met in the park, when Grace had been out walking the dog. I was taken aback as it was very unlike Grace to break through her natural reserve and make friends out of strangers. I had certainly never known her invite them into the house. It seemed that this might be the first sign that the disease was removing her natural inhibitions. The man must have been able to tell that I was not happy with the situation, and left soon after I arrived.

Once he had gone I asked Grace more about him, and she told me he was something to do with a religious order and was very knowledgeable about Scottish history, a subject dear to her heart. When I asked more questions she started to become agitated and confused, so I dropped the subject. Although I was happy there had been no wrongdoing this time, I was worried as to what might happen the next time Grace struck up a conversation with a complete stranger and invited him back to the house. I never saw the stranger again, and the phone calls stopped after that, so I assume they were from him.

Christopher had been in the house with her all the time that I had been away, but his life was now so separated and isolated from us and from the real world that I couldn't hope that he could be any support to his mother if anything ever went wrong. He certainly wouldn't have made any effort to ensure she was eating the right things, believing as he did that I was talking nonsense when I went on about diet being so important, and he wouldn't have worried if she invited a host of strange men into the house. Indeed it would have been consistent with his delusions about the security services and if she had done so he probably would have concluded that they were secret agents.

I knew I was going to have to be around to protect her and to do the cooking myself if I wanted to make sure that she was eating a decent diet of organic food, drinking spring water and taking her supplements. Just as she had once stayed home to look after the children when they were unable to fend for themselves, willing to suffer the financial penalties of not working, I had to find a way to be at home myself to look after her now that she needed me.

Christopher is by no means unusual in his scepticism about the importance of healthy eating. Some people believe that if they eat balanced diets they don't need any supplements, and it is certainly true that it is better for you to eat a diet of fresh food rather than fast food, but the food we buy from the supermarkets and call 'fresh' has still been grown in soils that

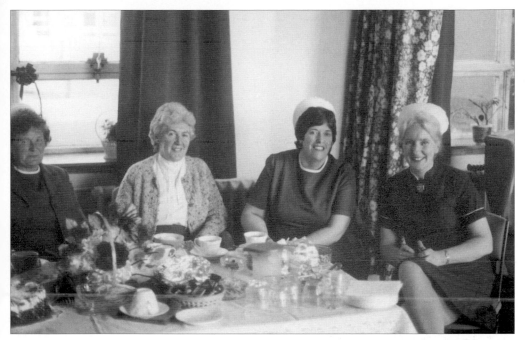

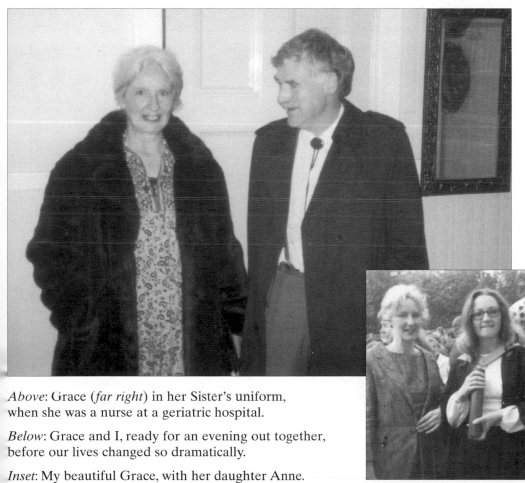

Above: Grace (*far right*) in her Sister's uniform, when she was a nurse at a geriatric hospital.

Below: Grace and I, ready for an evening out together, before our lives changed so dramatically.

Inset: My beautiful Grace, with her daughter Anne.

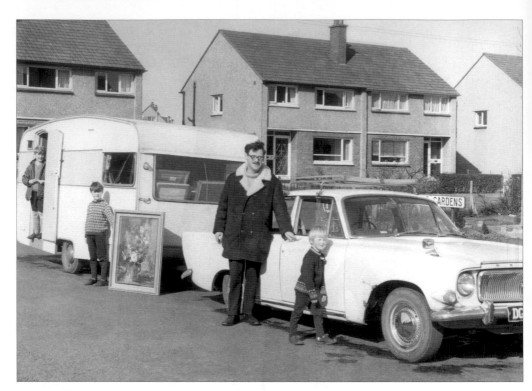

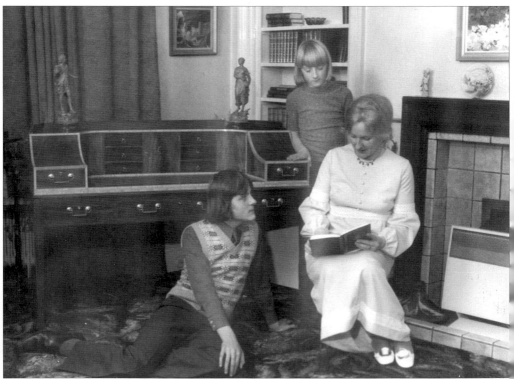

Above: Me, my sons and the mobile art gallery that was my business for many years.

Below: Grace with Kenneth (*sitting*) and Christopher, (*standing*). Tragically, Christopher went on to develop severe mental problems.

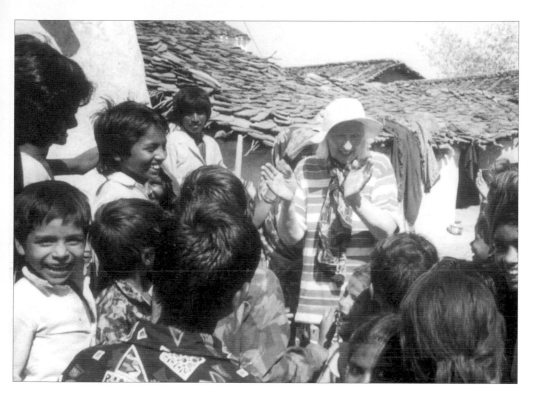

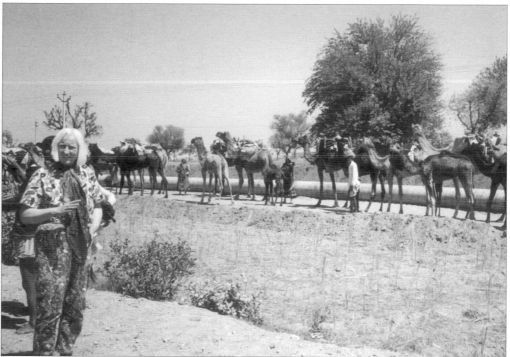

Above: Grace entertaining village children in India. Before the disease struck, she was a very reserved woman but one of the effects of the illness was her losing her inhibitions.

Below: Grace alongside a camel caravan in India.

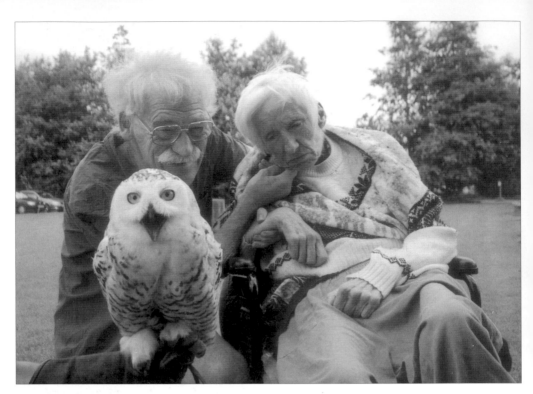

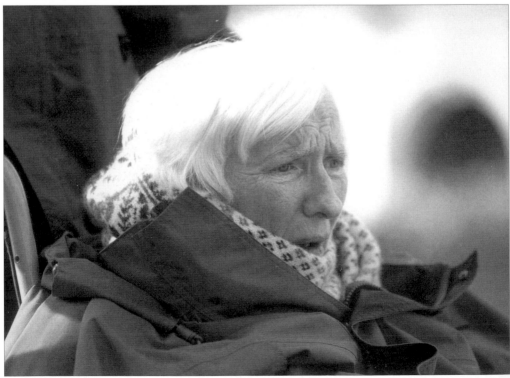

Above: Even when the disease was at a very advanced stage, I still did my best to stimulate Grace.

Below: A beautiful portrait of an incredible woman.

have been depleted through overworking, bad management and chemical fertilisers, and have then been enhanced with more chemicals to grow larger and to stay fresh-looking for longer. The next rung up the healthy-eating ladder are the foods described in the shops as being 'organic', meaning they have been produced without the aid of commercial and possibly poisonous fertilisers in the previous few years. That doesn't mean, of course, that the soil the organic crops are grown in is any richer in minerals than the soil that non-organic food is grown in. While we may be avoiding some of the toxins that pollute modern food by eating organically, we may still not be getting enough of the right vitamins and minerals, which is why supplements are still vital to maintain optimum health in the developed world.

Having said that, organic food is certainly a step in the right direction, and if farmers practise traditional farming methods for a number of years the condition of the soil should also improve, returning to the state it was in before we started to deplete it with modern farming methods. One study found that organic fruit and vegetables offered up to four times more trace elements than non-organic, thirteen times more selenium and twenty times more calcium and manganese. The organic foods that they studied also contained forty per cent less aluminium, twenty-nine per cent less cadmium, twenty-five per cent less lead and twenty-eight per cent less rubidium, all elements that are believed to contribute to disease. Non-organic foods contain a higher proportion of water, which makes them look plumper and more tempting but further dilutes the nutrients they contain.

Food isn't the whole story with Alzheimer's. There are a number of risk factors involved in all forms of dementia. The first is age, but there was nothing we could do about that one. The second is gender, with the male more likely to succumb than the female, so Grace had simply drawn the short straw on that one. High blood pressure is known to be a risk, and I was sure we could do something about that, as were coronary heart disease, diabetes and degenerative diseases of the arteries leading to a thickening of the arterial walls, and smoking. Anyone who has suffered from a stroke, embolism or thrombosis is also at risk of developing Alzheimer's.

In other words, an unhealthy lifestyle was very likely to make the situation much worse. Raised concentrations in the body of substances such as homocysteine are also risk factors in neuropsychiatric and thromboembolic disorders, and these can be effectively lowered with supplements of vitamin B6, vitamin B12 and folic acid.

I believe that once conventional medicine recognises the biochemical imbalance associated with dementia and works to correct it with mega doses of appropriate vitamins and minerals, then both sufferers and carers will be able to enjoy the same good, non-stressful lives that Grace and I embarked on as the disease took hold.

After bad diet, the next enemy we had to fight was stress. Stress, according to Dr Pfeiffer, produces dramatic biochemical changes within the body, and the longer it goes on, the greater the changes can be. At his clinic they have found, by testing hair, urine and blood samples to look for deficiencies, that when under stress individuals lose essential minerals such as potassium, calcium and zinc. They also tend to have high copper levels and, although a certain amount of copper is essential, too much can lead to acute depression. Stress can lead to people not sleeping properly, which leads in turn to more loss of important minerals. If the sleeplessness becomes chronic the missing minerals may never be made up in the body.

I needed to take drastic action if I wanted to ensure that Grace's life became stress-free and her diet became balanced. I could not control these things from a distance any longer. Just coping with the onset of the disease was stressful in itself, as was living with Christopher. I could no longer delay my decision; the business had to be disposed of, the bank repaid, the house in Glasgow sold and something more manageable found, so that I could concentrate my efforts on Grace's day-to-day needs.

Some of the pictures went back to the artists and I managed to do some sort of deal to get some money back. Others went up for auction and were sold at knockdown prices. The van also went, which meant that once I'd sold the house I would be able to repay the bank and I would still have enough to buy us somewhere smaller to live, hopefully leaving us with a cushion of a few thousand pounds for emergencies. It wasn't a great deal to show for all those years of work, but it was enough to ensure that we could live simply without having to worry about where the next penny was coming from.

Having put the house on the market, I went in search of somewhere new, something we could afford. The answer presented itself in Lanton, a hamlet about two miles down the hill from the town of Jedburgh, where a scattering of houses have been built on pretty, undulating farmland, about sixty miles south of Edinburgh, on the borders. Once the village had been able to boast three or four blacksmiths' premises, and there was a big house called Lanton Towers which looked as if it might once have been a fortified residence.

The Old School House, which was up for sale, was attached to a building that had once been a school but was now a village hall. There were enough rooms in the house for Christopher to have his own bedroom. The house had half an acre of garden, which we could use to grow some of the organic vegetables we needed to help us sustain a healthy life on a small budget. It was perfect and I made an offer that was accepted. We were on the move to our new life, my time entirely free to dedicate to the care of the wife who had looked after me so well for so many years.

I set to the task with enthusiasm, and once we'd moved in I did most of the gardening myself, despite the fact that I'd never had any experience and developed little aptitude for the work. Grace would always be at my side as I planted and watered and pruned and harvested our modest crops. I would find jobs for her to do that were within her capabilities, explaining to her over and over again how important her efforts were to the smooth running of our lives.

I'm sure that one of the most basic human needs is to believe that we are useful to others and effective in what we do. She always seemed to find contentment in the repetitive little jobs that we had to do amongst the fruit trees and vegetable plots, even if she would frequently forget what she was meant to be doing and wander off.

Eventually, when Grace needed continual watching and nursing, I did have to ask for the help of a gardener. There just weren't enough hours in the day to do all the jobs that needed doing if the crops were to be looked after and not allowed to go to waste, particularly if I had to keep breaking off from the task in hand in order to go after Grace and bring her back to somewhere safe.

I made sure we discussed and mutually agreed every job before we did it so that she would feel the deterioration of her household domain less acutely, and she would sometimes make wry little asides to visitors about my skills as a cook and house husband. I liked it when she teased me because it meant she still knew, most of the time, who I was, and remembered things about me. I knew that ability wouldn't last much longer.

If a job was obviously becoming too much for her I would politely ask if I could help her to complete it, and she was usually happy to hand it over, having grown frustrated with her own inability to get to grips with it. She could still easily be made to laugh at that stage, although that ability would also soon fade and her pretty face would stay sombre for longer and longer portions of the day.

I didn't get a phone installed in The Old School House as I thought the ringing would disorientate Grace, breaking the tranquillity of the house and making her anxious. It would also have been hard for me to concentrate my attention on her if I was constantly being interrupted by the demands of others. I wanted her to be the recipient of every second of my time. We didn't need to be in constant contact with the outside world by that stage anyway; the older children were busy with their own lives and seldom contacted us, and Christopher had no friends who would need to contact him. I found someone in the village who was willing to take messages for us, which we could pick up once a day when we were out walking.

Because Christopher had no work and no social life, leaving Glasgow wasn't a problem for him. He moved into his new downstairs bedroom with barely a word and hardly stirred from it, except for short, silent expeditions to the kitchen or the bathroom. He preferred to cook his own meals because he didn't trust us not to slip something into the food that he didn't want. In his demented world everyone was a potential enemy, even the people who had given birth to him and nurtured him through his childhood. He wanted no connection with us; he just required to be left alone. It tore me apart not to be able to help my son combat his illness in the same way that I helped Grace. But because of his paranoia, he was not receptive to my help, so all I could do was make sure he had a comfortable home and everything he needed. Once he was safely in behind his bedroom door he would put on Kylie Minogue CDs to pass the waking hours, or endlessly watch television programmes, safely separated from the real life outside the house, the life that caused him so much anxiety and unhappiness.

We still had a car when we first moved to Lanton, and were able to get into Galashiels once a week to buy the organic food and fresh oily fish that we wanted for our diet. I felt that it was as important for me to stay healthy as it was for Grace. If I became ill or worse, who would care for her then? The idea was too terrible to contemplate. I knew all the right things to do for her, so I must do them for myself as well.

We would usually get about five pounds of herring and mackerel, enough to last us until our next trip out. After shopping we would give ourselves a treat, making our way to a local café and having a gateau and a cup of coffee while the fishmonger gutted the fish we had selected. You can find so much pleasure in simple things when you look for it.

My cooking never became very fancy, but I was able to provide all the foods that Grace needed for her condition. The fresh fish that we bought I would fry in the evening with some organic oats. Now and then I would cook us a nice piece of steak. I would grind up all the vitamins and supplements that Grace needed and put them into crushed mango, papaya or banana to make them easy to swallow and digest.

Our days in The Old School House took on a peaceful routine. Even when the car had to go in order to save money, we kept up the shopping trips, using the local bus services. Getting on and off buses took a while as Grace lost the ability to climb steps, but other people were always very helpful and patient as I pushed from behind and guided her to a safe seat.

We'd bought a Border collie bitch to replace Meissen, and to begin with Grace was still able to go out of the house a little on her own, taking the dog with her to deter any strangers like the man in the Glasgow park. But when a neighbour complained that the dog had almost attacked his wife, I realised Grace had no control over it any more and that it wasn't safe to let her out on her own. From then on I thought we had better go out together.

A neighbour who had a male collie used to take our dog out for a walk sometimes and ours fell pregnant as a result. She had three puppies, which were fun for Grace to play with and which I managed to find homes for once they were old enough. The mother, unfortunately, became rather aggressive after that and went for Grace once or twice, perhaps alarmed by a noise she had made, or a sudden movement. Sadly, since I couldn't control the way Grace acted and I couldn't take the risk of anything worse happening, I had to get rid of the dog. It did at least mean one less distraction from the task of caring for Grace, which required more and more concentration with each passing day.

Other things were starting to go wrong for her as the effects of the disease crept inexorably onwards through her brain. She was beginning to lose the ability to do quite simple things, like wash herself or get to the toilet. The first time she wet herself, sitting in an armchair, she seemed to have no idea that it had happened. I realised that day that from then on I was going to have to take control of all her toilet habits, just as you would with a small child. I would have to make sure I took her into the bathroom every few hours and helped her to remove her clothes and sit down. By doing that I could keep her dry most of the day. If she did get wet, then I had to help her change into clean clothes. She would never know if she had had an accident so I had to be vigilant in case she sat for too long in wet clothes and became sore.

At night I would have to get her up a couple of times in order to take her to the toilet if I didn't want to wake up in the morning to find we had wet sheets. Often I would do this and she would still have had an accident before morning. I started putting plastic on the chair that she used to sit in next to the fire, and a plastic sheet on the bed to protect the mattress.

The people from the social services were very responsive to all my requests and provided us with gadgets to help me hoist Grace on and off the toilet and into the bath. I think they were anxious to encourage me to keep her at home for as long as possible. They needn't have worried; I had no intention of asking them to take over caring for her. That was my job.

I needed those gadgets as Grace became more confused because I wasn't able to lift her out of the bath once she was unable to help me herself. Getting in and out of a bath is a surprisingly complicated manoeuvre, nothing like just walking down a street or sitting in a chair, both of which she could still manage. If you think about how to do it, and which muscles to instruct to do what movement, you can appreciate that too much deterioration in the brain will make it impossible.

Often people with Alzheimer's become challenging, aggressive and difficult to handle, but Grace was always compliant and easy-going, if sometimes a little stubborn in the later stages. I was convinced that this tranquillity was partly, if not totally, because of the supplements and the diet. I also believed that as the disease grew worse she would need a calm, level and stable environment in which to thrive. Just as children with behavioural difficulties often behave beautifully as long as they are not hungry, wet, cold, hot, bored or unsettled in any way, I felt it was my job to make Grace's world both stimulating and tranquil, comfortable and safe.

As well as diet, the other element that I thought was critical both to her and me was exercise. I knew that exercise was one of the ways doctors advised people to cope with stress and I was determined that we should go for an eight-to-ten mile walk every day. If it was part of her routine, I reasoned, she would be happy to do it. It didn't matter how bad the weather might be – we had to get outside and take some exercise at least once a day. Not only was it good for us physically, it was also mentally very refreshing to look at the views and feel the breeze on our faces and our legs.

If the weather was reasonable, I would always take my shirt off to feel the air and the sun on as much of my skin as possible. It was a wonderful way to release any tensions. Imagine how it would have been if we had both been cooped up indoors together twenty-four hours a day with nothing to think about but the next trip to the bathroom – I think we would both have gone stir crazy within a week.

Walking is a tremendous way to take exercise because it is simple and pleasurable to do, requiring no special equipment or arrangements. Brisk walking, like structured exercise, can also prevent non-insulin-dependent (type II) diabetes. The ongoing Nurses' Health Study has shown that the brisker the walking pace, the lower the risk of developing diabetes. Others have found that it can improve heart health. Data from the nurses' study, based on 72,488 female nurses aged between forty and sixty-five, found that brisk walking for three or more hours lowered the risk of coronary heart disease by between thirty and forty per cent, the same reduction as seen with an hour-and-a-half of vigorous exercise per week.

This type of activity can also improve the functioning of the mind. When a team from the University of Illinois randomly assigned 124 sedentary adults aged between sixty and seventy-five to a programme of either brisk aerobic walking or non-aerobic stretching and toning exercises, they found that the walking group not only improved physically, but also experienced a clear improvement in cognitive function.

'Years ago, it was thought that rest and relaxation were the best ways to recuperate from injury or illness,' says Bengt Saltin, director of the Copenhagen Muscle Research Centre, 'but my research proved that, in fact, it is the opposite.' He made the discovery as part of a NASA-sponsored project looking at the effects of inactivity, confirming that exercise, not bed rest, should be a part of recovery. His studies of elite athletes while they are exercising and training have led to a better understanding of the regulation of oxygen flow to the muscles and the availability of nutrients in exercise and overall health.

Our excursions into the countryside, along paths edged with wild gorse and broom and fields dotted with wild orchids, gave the day a focus and filled some of the hours that we had together. In the morning I would be making our cheese sandwiches, so that we could have a snack while we were out. If wild berries were in season we would pick them – cherries, blackberries and raspberries – and eat them as we went. If the weather was wet I would cover our top halves in cagoules, but we would set out just the same.

About half a mile from the house was a river where swans cruised with their cygnets and where the wild ducks came in to roost in the evenings. Grace would clap her hands with delight as she watched them coming in to land and skidding across the water's surface like tiny waterskiers before settling down and restoring their dignity with a shake of their ruffled feathers.

Some of the neighbours told me later that they used to feel quite alarmed for us sometimes, seeing us several miles away from the house, trudging across a snowy or rain-swept field. But we were both very happy on our outings. I would hold her hand all the way, to guide her and stop her wandering off or sitting down, and we would talk about the views we were looking at from the hills, or the animals we were passing, or I would recite poems that I remembered, or sing songs.

One day the only word she could say was 'pink'. I asked her what colour she thought the trees were. 'Pink.' The hedges? 'Pink.' What colour is the sky? 'Pink.'

She never initiated any conversations, but she responded cheerfully to anything I brought up, even if her answer made little sense. Her talking became less and less frequent as the years went past, until she eventually fell completely silent, but I continued to tell her how beautiful she was and how much I loved her, sharing whatever plans I might have with her or describing what we were seeing out loud. Sometimes we would meet someone else on our walks and stop for a short conversation. I would ask those who didn't know her to say 'how are you?' to Grace, and just this simple question would sometimes find a surviving path of understanding through her brain and the enquirer would be rewarded with a charming smile and a twinkling eye. Everyone was always very kind and understanding.

Mr and Mrs Martin owned Lantonhill Farm, with its well-run kennels and dog obedience centre where labradors and spaniels were brought to be trained to the gun. Mrs Martin's father had died as a result of complications associated with Alzheimer's, so we were always sympathetically received there with a greeting and a word of encouragement. From Lantonhill Farm we would head over the hill, enjoying views along the way to Gospel Farm, which was once run by a religious group who were said to have met for worship under a tree that was struck by lightning. From there we turned into a country road and on down the main road to Bedrule, heading for the church, outside which was a seat for us to rest on and eat our sandwiches.

It was a pretty church, its stained-glass window depicting shepherds and sheep, as appropriate for the area. From our seat we could see across the river to the thousand-foot height of Rubislaw, one of the areas where I had spent so many years driving and camping with my dogs and my paintings. It was eight miles back to Bedrule, but sometimes we went on for another three or so miles after that. Grace would take a hundred deep breaths as she went, and talk to the sheep and cattle as we passed. These deep breaths were part of her treatment, and intended to combat the respiratory complaints that are often associated with Alzheimer's.

Sometimes, when we were out on our walks, she would just sit down in the road and refuse to get up. When that happened I wouldn't be strong enough to lift her on my own and I would have to enlist the help of anyone else who might be passing, whether that meant flagging them down in a car or knocking on someone's front door. No one ever turned down my requests for assistance.

Once we were home from our walks I would settle Grace down with a video of a musical and make her some tea. We tended to have fish on alternate days, with fresh meat (not chicken, as that didn't agree with Grace), eggs or cheese in between. By ten o'clock both of us were exhausted and ready for bed.

I felt that, even if Grace couldn't remember anything, there was no reason why I shouldn't make every moment of her life as interesting and comfortable as possible, even if that enjoyment was gone from her memory forever a few moments later.

Not very much happened in the village hall next door, apart from a Christmas party for the neighbourhood and sometimes a summer party with a barbeque when the eighty or so people of the village and outlying cottages would all get together. I put on an exhibition there, called 'Lanton 1996', and in the course of our walks Grace and I would ask everyone in the area if they had anything that we could use. About a third of them contributed something, whether it was a history of Lanton Towers or old agricultural equipment or paintings of the area. The Secretary of the Borough Council was very artistic and put it all together very nicely. People came from a wide area to look at it, and the newspapers and local radio stations showed a lot of interest.

It wasn't only when we were out on walks that Grace would occasionally stage sit-down strikes. Sometimes I would have to call on neighbours or flag down passers-by to help me lift her if she decided to sit down on the floor of the house or conservatory and not get up. Everyone was always very happy to help. It's surprising, once you're in that situation, how many other people you find have had experience of

Alzheimer's with their parents, partners or some other elderly relative. Anyone who has will always be very sympathetic to someone who is looking after another sufferer.

On one occasion we visited some friends of ours in Edinburgh, Frank and Elizabeth Girling, while they were having alterations made to the bathroom in their lovely Georgian house in Drummond Place. The building work meant I had to take Grace upstairs to the toilet, after which she refused to come back downstairs. It took us two hours to coax her down and at one stage we even considered calling the fire brigade and asking them to help.

There were other times when Grace would behave a little badly, but never for long. For a time she took to swearing rather a lot, something I never heard her do when she was still in control of what came out of her mouth. Her language would sometimes become particularly blue in the bathroom. I knew from my days as a nurse that the important thing was not to argue back when patients became belligerent, just to keep communicating through touches and smiles.

Sometimes she would refuse to do something I asked, like get up off some wet sheets. Unfortunately she did that one day when a welfare officer was coming to check how I was coping. They found her sitting on the wet bed at three in the afternoon being very grumpy indeed. They started to talk about referring her to a mental health team. The words frightened me because I couldn't imagine losing her to the care of anyone else or giving up the struggle against drugs. I knew from my own experience that once a patient like Grace was inside an institution they would administer sedatives the moment she was even slightly unco-operative. Whereas I had all the time in the world to wait for her to come round from a sulk, a busy nursing staff, with other patients to look after, was not likely to be willing to spend hours coaxing her to do what they wanted. Just as it is always easier to sit a troublesome child down in front of a television than to try to distract and stimulate him or her, it is always easier to sedate a patient than to humour them.

After the welfare officer had gone I chivvied Grace into drinking an extra-powerful nutritional cocktail and by the next morning she was back to her normal, gentle self and the welfare people decided to leave us alone for a bit longer.

Sometimes, when she could still talk, I would tease her, asking if she knew who I was – whether I was her husband or her fancy man. 'You're a rascal,' she would answer, with a twinkle in her eye. Eventually, of course, the twinkle died and she said nothing to any of the questions anyone put to her.

At the suggestion of the welfare officer I took Grace to a day centre one day, leaving her for just four-and-a-half hours in order to get a little time to myself, but she was in floods of tears all the time because she thought I'd deserted her, so I didn't repeat the exercise for many years.

CHAPTER EIGHT

The Food of Love

Music, when soft voices die,
Vibrates in the memory.
PERCY BYSSHE SHELLEY

As well as a good diet and exercise, I believed that music and love were also important ingredients in Grace's routine – vital tools to soothe the soul as well as the mind.

Now that I had more time to reflect back over our life together I was afraid that I might have been an ungenerous lover in the many years of our marriage. The incident of the erotic book she had placed on my desk kept rising involuntarily to my thoughts and I found myself wondering increasingly often what had gone through Grace's mind at the time to make her do something so out of character. I hadn't had the courage to ask her at the time and it was far too late to ask her now, when she couldn't remember what had happened a few moments before, let alone a few years.

But I remembered the incident clearly, and it was troubling

me. Ever since our stolen hours in the doctors' quarters at St Giles Hospital, I never ceased to find her attractive and desirable. But I now knew I had never really taken enough care about ensuring she had enjoyed herself before I fell asleep with her in my arms.

I wondered, now, how often she must have lain awake, aroused by our love-making and unsatisfied by its conclusion, while I slept like a dead man. One of the main platforms of the women's movement, if the glossy magazines of the time were to be believed, was that women were as entitled to enjoy sexual activity as men, and I wondered if she read those articles and tried to think of ways to broach the subject with me delicately, without offending me. I'd like to think that if she had brought the subject up I would have had the courage and decency to listen to what she had to say and act upon it but, if that was the case, why did I not respond to the hint of that carefully placed book with its clear and well-illustrated message? It seemed likely that I would not have responded well to criticism in this area, and Grace was never one to introduce any notes of discord into our relationship if she could help it. Would she have lived a more pleasurable married life if I had been a little more concerned about her welfare in this respect? That was the thought that plagued me now.

All these questions troubled my conscience and I wanted to make amends in any way I could before it was too late. I wanted to ensure that Grace received all the pleasure I was capable of giving her now that her well-being was my one and only concern. More importantly, however, I was certain that sexual satisfaction would help her to achieve serenity in the difficult years she was facing, and so I was intent on finding ways of achieving it for her.

People with dementia often undergo massive personality changes and wild mood swings, becoming depressed and anxious one moment, euphoric the next. They lose their inhibitions, which can be alarming for all those around them until they grow used to it. They are often agitated, apathetic or irritable. They can also suffer from hallucinations, delusions and even eating disorders. It is when they are confronted with all these ominous-sounding possibilities that many carers panic, believe they can't cope and immediately book their poor relatives into institutions. But not all these things have to happen if you are careful. In fact, you may be able to avoid all of them if you do everything possible to achieve serenity for the patients.

Now that I was spared the distraction of earning a living, I felt that I could pay Grace back a little for all her quiet, patient support down the years, with more time and attention. When you don't have to rush off to work every day you can put a lot of hours into other parts of your life.

Our routine, once we moved to The Old School House in Lanton, grew regular. Every morning we would wake up naturally at about seven o'clock. I would make sure that Grace was in the mood for a cuddle, which she usually was and then. I would help her to get up and into the bathroom where I would give her a shower. I would try to make it fun for her, as the more she enjoyed herself, the less likely it was that she would become difficult and obstructive in the washing process.

If she didn't feel like a cuddle when she first woke up and grumbled or pushed me away, we would go to the shower first and that would usually make her more relaxed. Sometimes she would be a little agitated and angry in the bathroom, swearing and shouting at whatever shadows were passing through her mind, but by the time we were coming out of the bedroom for breakfast she would be as gentle and relaxed as a lamb.

When we first arrived at The Old School House I bought a little conservatory in a sale, which I erected on the side of the garage where it would catch the sun and where there was a good view of the garden. Four apple trees stood on one side and a rose garden on the other with a hedge behind it, masking the small road, and fields beyond where the farmer would bring his rams to rest after they had done their work with the ewes. It was a very pretty, tranquil spot.

Once I had got Grace dressed, which could take quite a long time if she wasn't in the mood to co-operate, I would lead her out to the conservatory, make her comfortable in her favourite chair and ready for a breakfast of fruit and cereal. By this time I was having to feed her like a baby, since she found the job of operating cutlery and getting food from the plate to her mouth herself impossible. It would take a little while to coax each spoonful between her lips, but there was no hurry – we had all morning.

I would then turn our old Marconi radio on to Classic FM, which was her favourite station. The music soothed her and she would sit listening quietly while I went indoors to the kitchen and prepared the sandwiches for our daily walk. I'm sure that the music made it through into her brain in ways the spoken word no longer did, the rhythms signalling to her in some primitive way that everything in the universe was as it should be and that there was no reason for her to be angry or worried about anything. Music even seemed to remain in her memory when everything else had slipped away, and often she would be humming or singing remembered tunes as she wandered vacantly through the day, unable to piece together even a simple sentence of words.

Not everyone liked the idea of Grace and me still having an active sex life in our situation, but I was always very open about it. I was – and remain – quite certain that it was beneficial for Grace, and I believe that other Alzheimer's sufferers would definitely benefit from a similar regime. One day, a few years later, I discussed the subject at a monthly meeting of carers at the day hospital to which I would take Grace once a week towards the end of her life. I think the idea of the meeting was for us all to have a crying session because they provided tissues as we came into the room, but I never felt like crying. I was always too busy and too happy.

About eight of us were sitting in a circle and, as often happened when I had extended conversations with people about what my life with Grace was like, I talked about our love life. I have always found it an easy subject to talk about, even though I know other people aren't necessarily as comfortable as I am with the concept.

It seems to be the generally accepted view that sufferers of

Alzheimer's do not, and should not, have active sex lives, even if they are in happy and long-lasting relationships with their carers. It's a view I strongly disagree with and I said so. I could tell I was getting a bit of a mixed reaction.

The next thing I knew, the sister in charge of the day hospital and the community psychiatric nurse who worked with her were knocking on our front door later that day, asking if they could come in for a chat. I was always happy to have familiar faces dropping in on Grace. I thought it made a pleasant distraction for her and wished that more of our old friends and family felt they could do the same. Sadly, the majority of the world preferred to leave us to our own devices by that stage, particularly those who had once been closest to Grace.

Once the two ladies were settled down comfortably in the conservatory they told me that they wanted to have a chat with me about what I had been discussing at the day centre, because it had made some people uncomfortable. They were both very nice ladies who knew us well and had been extremely helpful in settling us into our new house. They were apologetic, and told me that they knew how well I cared for Grace and that she was one of the most tranquil and satisfied Alzheimer's sufferers they had ever come across. They were aware that I had never made any secret of our continuing love life and was not being furtive about it. I felt rather sorry for them since they seemed to have been put in a deeply embarrassing position.

After they'd asked whatever questions they had come to ask,

and had enjoyed a cup of tea with us, they went away to report back their findings. Later that day the psychiatric nurse stopped by again just to let me know that they were perfectly happy that Grace couldn't be better cared for. It was kind of her to take so much trouble to put my mind at ease, because I knew that if things went wrong it was very possible they could separate Grace from me and I would have the devil of a job to get her back once she had been assimilated into the bureaucratic system.

I can understand why people would be concerned. There was no way in the final years of her life that Grace could have been said to be able to give consent for me to have sex with her, although I was always confident that until the last few months she was capable of showing me that she didn't welcome my attentions by pushing me away or shouting out.

Just as she was unable to give clear consent, however, she was also unable to withhold it. So how do you judge whether or not it was the right thing to do? She couldn't consent to being fed, or washed or taken to the toilet either, but no one would have suggested for a moment that I should assume she didn't want any of those things to happen.

I could quite understand that it was not as straightforward a moral issue as I might have believed in the earlier stages of the illness, and some people would say that to be on the safe side I should simply have put a stop to our sex life as soon as the disease took hold. My argument to that is that I am certain Grace enjoyed the physical attention of being stroked and petted. She was indisputably calmer and more contented than most Alzheimer's patients, and I believe strongly that her sexual satisfaction contributed to that state, although there is no way that I can ever prove it.

If a carer is the sufferer's lifetime partner, then I think they have to be trusted to make the right decisions unless there is obvious evidence of physical abuse or emotional distress which could be traced back to the sexual activity. I realise, however, that there will be some readers who will strongly disagree and others who would just prefer not to think about the whole issue.

CHAPTER NINE

TRAVELLING
WITH GRACE

So then Dr Froyd said that all I needed was to
cultivate a few inhibitions and get some sleep.

ANITA LOOS IN GENTLEMEN
PREFER BLONDES

O nce we were settled into The Old School House in Lanton
and our retirement had taken on a steady rhythm, I
began to think again about travelling, remembering the many
places Grace and I had been to before the illness struck, and
the many experiences we had enjoyed.

Although I was very happy with our simple life in the
Scottish countryside, I missed the stimulation of seeing new
places and learning about new cultures. I was beginning to
wonder if there was any reason why we shouldn't now do a
little more travelling together. Grace's illness would be with us
whether we were walking across windswept Scottish fields or
sun-drenched Caribbean beaches, but the latter might offer
her some benefits that the former could not, as well as offering
me a break from the routine of home life.

Why, I reasoned, now that we had endless amounts of time on our hands, should we not go abroad and see some of the places we had always dreamed of seeing? If we didn't do it soon it was quite possible that in a few years one or other of us would not be able to do it at all, and we would have missed our opportunity. I have always been a great believer in seizing whatever opportunities life offers – and we were being offered a great deal of leisure time.

By the mid-nineties, Christopher had become too much for me to be able to handle at home. He was in and out of hospital all the time and needed more or less constant professional supervision by trained community psychiatric social workers. I had to admit to myself that I couldn't look after both him and Grace. I felt that my first allegiance had to be to Grace, particularly since she needed and wanted my help, whereas Christopher was openly rejecting it.

If my first duty was to my wife, then I was going to have to hand over responsibility for my son to someone else. Neither of his brothers or his sister wanted anything to do with him, or he with them, so the local authorities found him a flat where he could live when he was out of hospital and where they could keep an eye on him to ensure that he did not reach a pitch of depression where he might be tempted to try suicide again.

His life didn't change much – he simply moved from living in one room to living in another. I dare say that he was as relieved to be away from us as I was to be away from him. A young lad with a car would come to the flat and take him out once a week to get whatever shopping he needed, and the doctors would try to keep him stable on drugs. I still believed there must have been alternative ways of treating the illness, but if neither Christopher nor his doctors wanted to follow that route there was nothing I could say or do. In a way I did feel that I was letting him down by handing over the responsibility for my son to someone else, but I had to accept that there were limits to what I could do. He hardly acknowledged us at all any more, and never wanted us to visit him when he was in hospital. He had become a stranger to the whole family and I had to accept that there was nothing more I could achieve. I had to concentrate my efforts on giving Grace as nice a life as possible.

Our financial situation had settled down for the first time in our lives. With the small amounts of money we had put aside over the years for pensions, we had enough to support ourselves with just a bit to spare. I could see no reason why I wouldn't be able to look after Grace in other places just as well as I was doing in Lanton – and life in warmer climates is almost always cheaper when you don't need to worry about heating bills.

The choices open to us seemed to be either to sit in Lanton and wait for the disease to grow worse and for Grace to eventually die, or to go out looking for a bit of fun and excitement. I decided on the latter, and we set off, our luggage clanking with Grace's pills and with a tape machine to play her favourite music wherever we might end up.

We started with a trip to Italy, a country we had been to

before and to which I had always vowed I would return when I had more time to spend there. We left England for Florence in the early spring, before the tourist season got under way and before the heat became too intense, and stayed in youth hostels and cheap boarding houses along the way.

It was blissful. Instead of taking our afternoon walks across the Scottish countryside we strolled round the many galleries, churches and palaces together, with me giving Grace running commentaries as we went and her smiling sweetly and taking none of it in, just gazing at the pictures before shuffling on, sometimes clapping her hands or making little noises of appreciation or excitement. It sounded to me like she was enjoying herself. There are some advantages to growing old, and most of the places we wanted to see we could get into free, just by showing our passports and proving that we were retired.

For any lover of art and lover of life Florence is a magical city. The youth hostel we found there was a beautiful old house set in some woods on the outskirts of the city, full of carved marble statues and big, cool, stone-floored rooms. There was a rumour that it had once been the home of Mussolini's mistress. The managers gave us a family room, which meant we had our own bathroom and didn't have to queue up with other guests or worry about the noises Grace might make while I was struggling to wash her or when she was sitting on the toilet.

In the restaurant there was always a choice of two meals, so we used to order one of each and then share them, me feeding both of us and talking for both of us at the same time. I would allow myself a glass or two of wine, although Grace would not drink alcohol. In the mornings, after a breakfast of rolls and cocoa, we would stroll through the woods in the warm spring sunshine or catch a bus down into the centre of town, where all the art was waiting for us, as were the shady back streets and the piazzas with their bakeries and coffee shops.

What I like about staying in hostels is that there are so many younger people around. They were always more relaxed in their attitudes towards Grace, unworried by her behaviour, amused by her and happy to talk to her as if she could understand everything they said. I remember on a later trip, when we were crossing a border in South America somewhere, a group of helpful students lifted her bodily on to the top of a cart carrying all the rucksacks and luggage, giving her a joyful ride past the laughing border guards.

Young travellers would always be willing to help us on and off trains or buses, and talk to us at meal times. I think travelling has that effect on people. It puts them in a good mood and, because they're not on their own territory, travellers don't feel threatened by someone different and unpredictable. They have time to spare and an openness to new ideas and experiences that they might not have when they are back in their home countries.

In a way we already lived in a different land to the young. When you are nineteen and in full health, with your whole life spread out in front of you, you can't believe you belong to the same species as those who are nearing the end of their lives and are speaking the language of dementia. Watching me feeding Grace at the dinner table must have seemed as distant to their daily experience as the times when their mothers did the same for them. For people who were nearer our own age it must have been a more disturbing sight, a chilling reminder of how close to the edge we all are and how easily we can wake up to find we have stepped over to the other side, moving in a few short strides from normality to insanity.

After a couple of weeks in Florence we caught a bus to Siena where we stayed in a nunnery, in a room overlooking the old town, beyond which was a cathedral that was lit up at night, giving us a spectacular view. The nuns didn't provide food but there was a wonderful little restaurant nearby, full of local people who were happy to welcome us into their midst every evening as they settled down to eat and talk and laugh.

From there we moved on to Assisi and Rome for more galleries and sights. I remember one painting in particular that struck me as very moving. There was an angel floating above and putting her hand down to a little boy, her other hand pointing upwards. I assumed the little boy had died and was being taken to heaven. We stood together, hand in hand, staring up at it for a long time.

From Rome we caught a train to Sicily, which was carried across the water on a boat, depositing us on the dockside. We stayed in the cliff-top village of Taormina, where every house seemed to be covered in fragrant spring blossoms which had not yet been battered and bleached by the heat of high summer, and climbed Mount Etna, although the tour guides wouldn't let Grace too close to the rim in case she stumbled on the rough shingle.

We took boats to the outer islands where all the locals who had rooms to let were gathered at the docks, waiting for us, jabbering their offers and beckoning us to follow them rather than their neighbours. We were led to a flat by an eager old woman who talked to us non-stop all the way, and we stayed with her for a week or so. We took lovely long walks in the sun and boat trips round the islands. We saw the volcano on Stromboli glowing against the night sky, and bathed in dark, therapeutic mud on Volcano Island before washing off in volcanic springs. I could see that being in the warmth after the long Scottish winter was helping Grace to relax. As she unwound I thought I spotted fleeting glimpses of her old self.

On the way back up Italy by train we disembarked at the bustling railway station in Naples. As I tried to sort out Grace and the luggage, a man working as part of an organised gang grabbed my rucksack, in which I kept all our money and travel documents, and made a run for it. I'd been warned so often that this sort of thing would happen in Italy, but I was still caught off guard, my mind busy with other problems. I knew that I had to get the bag back; there simply wasn't an option. I had to leave a confused-looking Grace, surrounded by our few other pieces of luggage, and run after the thief.

Thank goodness I'd been taking so much exercise over the previous few years because he was a good deal younger than me. I caught up with him before he got off the station concourse and snatched the bag back. I think he must have been surprised to have been chased by an old man, because he made no attempt to fight over it, just vanished into the crowd as I made my way quickly back to Grace, who was still standing where I'd left her, gazing around in blissful ignorance of the whole episode.

It wasn't the last time that we would be the victims of bag-snatchers – I guess we were bound to look like an easy target to any thieves working in crowded, tourist-filled areas – but I always managed to get our property back before it disappeared forever.

We made our way up Italy to Venice and then on back to England. The whole trip lasted nearly three months and, having returned home successfully, I knew that it wouldn't be long before we would be off somewhere new. I had discovered that what might once have seemed impossible was in fact perfectly possible. Once we had got past the difficult part of deciding to do it, travelling hadn't been difficult at all.

When we arrived at any establishment that we wanted to stay in, I had to let them know that there might be trouble with bed-wetting. They were always very understanding and willing to send sheets to the laundry each day if necessary. Later I discovered the wonders of adult nappies or incontinence pads, which would keep Grace comfortable for up to six hours at a time and save on all the laundry problems. I wished I'd discovered them years before. It was much easier to lay her down and change her just like a baby every few hours than trying to coax her into toilets when she might not want to go, particularly in public places.

At the time of the Italian trip she was still very well behaved and no trouble to anyone. On subsequent trips she would sometimes become a little too noisy in the hotel rooms, and once or twice we were asked to leave places because she was disturbing the other guests with her shouting in the night. The problem was that the places we were staying in were always the cheapest I could find, which meant that sometimes the walls were paper-thin or the doors didn't fit particularly well, and so there was no soundproofing. I suppose that some of the noises Grace would make from time to time would have sounded a little disturbing if heard coming out of the stillness of the night. I was used to them and never thought anything of them, just that they were part of the way she was, but I could understand why other people might be made uncomfortable by them, imagining something awful might be happening on the other side of their bedroom walls.

There was never any point in protesting or arguing if someone had made a complaint about us to the management. If the managers asked us to leave we would always do so, and we always seemed able to find somewhere else where they were more accommodating before nightfall. The managers were nearly always very sad to have to ask us to leave, although once or twice they became angry with Grace, seeming to think that she was doing it on purpose, and my language skills were not good enough to be able to explain to them that she had no more idea about the sounds she was making than she did about anything else.

Getting on to aircraft could sometimes be difficult, if Grace was acting up in the airport. It tended to happen most if there were delays and she was kept hanging about too long in the terminal and became uncomfortable and fidgety. We were only actually turned back at the gate once, in Mexico, when the staff felt that she wasn't safe to fly. We came back the next day, when Grace was calmer, and had no trouble getting her on board.

Almost as soon as we got back to Lanton after the first trip to Italy, I started laying plans for the next year. I thought this time we would go to Northern India, visiting Delhi, Jaipur, Agra, Gwalior, Orchha, Khajuraho, Varanasi and Lucknow. This time it seemed like a better idea to take an organised tour. It was going to cost much more money, but I didn't feel as confident of finding my own way around India as I had in Italy. We still had some savings and I wanted Grace to see the beautiful architectural sights while she was still able to appreciate them, if only for a few moments at a time. It probably wasn't a wise use of our last savings, but we got to stay in some of the most splendid old hotels, including the guesthouse of a Maharajah, which looked as if nothing much had changed since the Raj left. Hotel gardens were filled with flowers like Dahlias, Hollyhocks and Sweet William, the swimming pools surrounded with colour. Bougainvillea and Flame of the Forest grew wild everywhere. We went on safari in a jeep and saw monkeys, antelopes and many other wild animals. There were crocodiles in the river and we got thoroughly filthy from the dust and dirt. We visited a wild bird nature reserve, where we saw species I'd never heard of before, as well as beautiful great eagles, which soared above us as we were quietly punted along waterways in a flat-bottomed boat. We rode elephants up to Amber Fort and we saw the sun rise on the Ganges. We visited some tenth-century Hindu erotic stone carvings at Khajuraho. We saw the magnificent Taj Mahal.

I still have hundreds of pictures in my mind from those wonderful days that I can savour whenever I care to, and I just hope that Grace got some pleasure from watching the scenes flicker past her before they disappeared into the blackness where her memory had once been. When you have no memory, life and experience take on completely different meanings. In a way Grace was behaving more naturally than I, like an animal or a bird or a fish, just enjoying what was happening to her with no thought of the past or the future. It was me who was confusing things by intellectualising them with meaningless concepts like remembrance and planning, imagination and interpretation. Eventually my mind too will stop working and all the images that I hold in storage will disappear for good, just as surely as they escaped from Grace, like a box full of old holiday photographs consigned to the bin during an attic clearout.

India was a great experience, and the people we met were all sweetly accepting of Grace. Sometimes in the street, having lost all her inhibitions to the disease, she would start to play up a bit and a crowd of delighted children would gather round for the performance. The more they laughed and applauded, the more she would wave her arms about in a strange dance of her own, her face expressionless, an enigma. Sometimes I could see that other people on the tour were a touch embarrassed by the attention Grace attracted to us. It was impossible to imagine that this colourfully dressed, comical figure was the same person as the quiet, reserved, ladylike girl that I'd met and married all those years before.

It's funny how easily people are embarrassed by adults behaving in an uninhibited manner. If a small exuberant child started dancing in the street, clapping their hands and twirling around, none of us would feel threatened. In fact, we would most likely be enchanted by the sight, finding it life enhancing to watch such *joie de vivre* and exchanging knowing smiles with one another. But, when an adult, particularly an elderly one, behaves in exactly the same way, many of us cringe and avert our eyes. It goes against all the conditioning that went into turning us into well-mannered, responsible adults. It's considered bad form to act irrationally and unpredictably. Children have no such inhibitions. If someone is being funny they will laugh, if they are acting strangely they will watch in awe, curious to know what will happen next.

It was hard to keep Grace on her diet in India, since she wasn't supposed to eat either chicken or rice, both of which turn up at just about every meal in that part of the world, but we survived with a bit of ingenuity. I consoled myself with the thought that most of what we did eat was probably organic as the majority of Indian agriculture seemed not to use fertilisers or pesticides and was better balanced than western systems. Whatever problems we might have with diet were more than compensated for by the benefits of the sunshine, warm air and constant stimulation.

CHAPTER TEN

SEEKING THE SUN

Mother, give me the sun.

HENRIK IBSEN

The following year we went to southern India, and this time I felt experienced enough to organise the trip myself, helped by a Lonely Planet guidebook and travelling once more amongst the young and a few other ageless hippies like ourselves, rather than the better-heeled folk who can afford the tailored packages and prefer to be separate from people as unpredictable as my Grace.

We couldn't have afforded another package experience anyway, however pleasant it might have been. Left to our own devices, and making the itinerary up as we went along, as we had in Italy, we stayed in all sorts of places, including one extremely basic hotel on the beach, where all the rooms were open to the elements. It was very cheap, and you had to go to bed with your money firmly attached to your person if you didn't want to lose it while you slept.

Where Grace was at a disadvantage when it came to remembering all the wonderful sights and experiences, she was at a decided advantage when it came to forgetting the inevitable disasters along the way that every traveller has to endure at some stage of any trip that is remotely adventurous. There were sometimes problems with finding clean water that Grace could use to take her tablets or to wash properly, and in one place she got painful mosquito bites. I got bitten as well, but mine didn't turn septic as hers did.

I tried to bandage Grace's raw-looking legs to protect them from any further infection, but I could tell after a few days that I needed medical help and checked her into a hospital. There they were very understanding and gave her some penicillin to clear up the infection before we travelled on to Sri Lanka, where we visited the baby-elephant sanctuary before going to Colombo, the capital city.

As we sat in the shade of the jungle growth watching the animals cavorting in the water, Grace's eyes wide with excitement, I knew that she had no memory at all of the unpleasant few days she had spent in the hospital ward. Life for her was strictly for the moment, and at that moment it had become wonderful once more.

Things were still very unsettled politically in Sri Lanka. There were roadblocks everywhere, and I was a little nervous that Grace might let off a strange noise at a tense moment and startle one of the many armed men who stopped us and inspected the occupants of the coach, but we made it to the city safely. A few weeks after we left the country a bomb went off in one of the temples we had visited, reminding me what a volatile world we all live in.

With our interest in diet and supplements, we had been able to perfect a formula for avoiding diarrhoea and sickness while travelling through unfamiliar lands and eating unfamiliar foods. During all of Grace's travels, she never once had trouble with her stomach, which made my life amongst the nappies a great deal easier. The formula was remarkably simple. Starting one month before travel, and continuing until you return from abroad, take daily: 2g vitamin C with bioflavonoids; 1 one-a-day Kwai concentrated garlic tablet; 1 one-a-day cod liver oil capsule.

Having discovered the *Lonely Planet* guides there was no stopping us. After returning from our second visit to India we took several trips to Cuba, each lasting a couple of months, where we were enchanted by the salsa music that seemed to be seeping out of every building and playing on every street corner, and where natives shinned up trees to cut down coconuts for Grace to drink the milk. We would go walking in the mornings and then get a meal in the evening, listening to the music of the streets. Some evenings I would organise picnic suppers on the beach to save a few more dollars; the local dogs would sit around us, patient and polite, waiting to be invited. One evening they were joined by a couple of pigs, whose manners were not so delicate, and we were forced to make a hasty escape.

Life was very cheap in Cuba, and we could get into

wonderful concerts for next to nothing. The seas were perfect for Grace, warm, calm and shallow, so she could play without any danger. Swimming was another way that she took exercise. In the sixth or seventh year of the disease she received her 'double channel challenge' certificate for swimming forty-two miles at Galashiels public swimming pool in one year.

In the course of our travels we followed the golden road to Samarkand, Bukhara and Tashkent, attended musical performances in one-time Islamic temples and courtyards where swifts would circle our heads while the music played. At a crocodile farm in India Grace held a young crocodile in her hand, her eyes wide with wonder. We stayed in cabins in the rain forest with only mesh-covered windows between us and the passing wildlife. We listened to the cacophony of jungle sounds at Tikal, a famous Maya site in Guatemala. The wealth of sights and sounds that the world has to offer was overwhelming, and at times I felt as removed from reality as Grace, no more than an audience to the earth's endless pageant.

When we discovered South America it felt like coming home, as if the whole continent had just been waiting for us to discover that this was where we belonged. We wandered around Peru, Mexico, Ecuador and the Galapagos Islands, loving everything about the place, staying for six months at a time and spending as little as five dollars a day on accommodation. We passed the evenings listening to the pipes and strings of the local musicians, instruments that we were able to try for ourselves at the Musical Museum in La Paz,

Bolivia, making Grace giggle and squeak with delight. We travelled over bumpy roads with the locals on their hot, crowded, noisy buses in order to save money and make the trips last longer.

One morning in Aguas Calientes, staying at Gringo Bill's guesthouse, I woke early. As Grace was still fast asleep I decided not to wake her and went out to the thermal spring swimming pool for a little time on my own. In the baths I met the director of the British Council in La Paz, a Scotsman from the Mull of Kintyre, who was on a motorcycling holiday with a beautiful young Bolivian girl. He told me he had seen Grace being helped down from Machu Picchu. When we were next in La Paz we dropped in to visit him, but he came out to tell us he was too busy to see us so we repaired to the café instead.

On the Galapagos Islands we visited the Charles Darwin Research Station where scientists are studying all sorts of life forms, including the famous giant tortoises of the islands. I fell into conversation with them about one tortoise in particular, known as Lonely George, who was only about a hundred and ten years old but who seemed to have lost interest in females. This was a subject very dear to my heart, and I suggested that they give him plenty of zinc and other minerals to build up his sex drive!

The islands were about as close to paradise as you can get, despite the heat, with sharks so friendly you could swim amongst them, snakes in the gardens that carried no poison and mosquitoes that bit but bore no malaria. Beautiful, colourful birds seemed unafraid of people, and iguanas, multicoloured crabs and lizards would sit next to Grace on the beach without fear.

I loved being in Lima, going to the South American Explorers' Club where you can study the area, and all the museums where you can see so much of the culture. The club's walls were draped in maps, which shimmered with the light breeze from the open windows and overhead fans. The eager young staff members were happy to help Grace up and down stairs, and provided her with a snake-embroidered, bamboo-cushioned chair. It was the perfect place for reading, making notes and meeting the many, mainly young people who were so pleased to relate stories of their adventures.

I particularly remember the exhibits at the Gold Museum, as well as the excellent coffee and orange cake that they served to visitors in the café. The museum has a large basement full of thousands of gold pieces from various cultures, and beautiful ceramics, especially of the Mochica period which dates from AD 0–700, including many exquisite pieces depicting human erotica.

The journey up to Cusco and Machu Picchu had to be broken for about ten days in Arequipa to allow for acclimatisation in preparation for the more rarefied atmosphere of Cusco. Arequipa has almost a million inhabitants and is 2,325 metres above sea level. It is a beautiful city surrounded by spectacular mountains, including the volcano, El Misti.

Grace and I stayed in a matrimonial room in the safe Hostel Santa Catalina, which is run by young male Jehovah's Witness students. They made us welcome and comfortable, meeting and helping us on and off our buses at the beginning and end of each day.

Close by the hostel there is the atmospheric Santa Catalina monastery. A few hundred years ago it inspired the lives of the daughters of the rich who attended for religious study and social intercourse, accompanied by their servants. Grace enjoyed seeing the small domestic units in which the girls lived. We spent a few hours getting the feel of the monastery by rambling through the narrow streets of its extensive ecclesiastical domain.

In Arequipa's museum we saw the preserved bodies of some of the Inca girls who were sacrificed to pacify the El Misti volcano; the girls had to be young, beautiful virgins. They were educated and proud of their role in the preservation of the people. They had to trudge up the mountain in their sandals and at the top they drank their final sleeping potion before being battered to death. Large clots were visible in the brains of some of the bodies, evidence of how violently they had died. The dead girls had been preserved in the snow for around five hundred years, and were only uncovered recently when hot ashes from a nearby erupting volcano melted the snow and the bodies slid down the mountainside.

The road from the monastery leads into the central square or *Plaza de Armas*. On the left is the cathedral and on the right stand offices and a pleasant café serving the best coffee I've ever tasted. Sitting outside with a large pot in front of her, Grace was guaranteed always to attract a crowd with her antics.

Whilst in Arequipa we took a trip to the Valley of the Condors, staying overnight in a small town and bathing in a swimming pool filled from the warm thermal springs. A pretty local girl in our party, well contoured, coloured and boobed, mystified us by bouncing up and down in the water! That evening we watched a performance of music and dance based on Andean folklore while partaking of Peruvian mountain food. A lady, wild and weird, showed us to our accommodation, where we slept.

Next day, we arose early to enjoy breathtaking views along the hazardous roads as we travelled to the Valley of the Condors. The large and beautiful birds took our breath away as they came into view, soaring amongst the awe-inspiring mountains, which stretch up to heights of over 20,000 feet. In the valleys below, natives work just as the Incas did five hundred years ago, oblivious to the frantic pace of change in other parts of the world.

We bought some tasty local fruits from roadside sellers, and stopped at a dairy for the best cheese I have ever had. We passed poorly dressed local Indian people who appeared to be an integral part of this rugged and beautiful environment high up in the Andes. At the end of the day we returned to our hostel and ate at a Krishna restaurant.

I could see that, each time we came back to Scotland from a warm climate, Grace was finding it harder and harder to cope with the cold. With the sun on her she seemed to blossom, but in the chill and wet of the Scottish winters her petals would curl up again and she would go even further back inside herself until I could get her back to the warmth.

I was so enchanted by the whole atmosphere of South America that in 2000 I decided we should sell up in Lanton, since we were only there for about half the year anyway, and move to Peru permanently, so that Grace could end her days in the warm, with enough money to live a little more comfortably. We would be able to visit spas every day, eat in nice little local fish restaurants and breathe the clear mountain air. I suppose it was a foolish dream, but then many people would have said it was a foolish idea to take Grace travelling in the first place, and that had worked out well. And others would have said I was stupid to have taken on nursing her myself, but I certainly never regretted that.

In my opinion it never does any good to listen to others when they suggest that you shouldn't do things, or when they tell you that things you want to do will be beyond your capabilities. They are bound to be right now and then, but think of all the times they will be wrong and you will have missed out on something wonderful by taking heed of their warnings. I had made up my mind that it was time to move from Scotland to Peru.

Robert Bathgate, a neighbour of ours in Lanton, was six years old when his mother asked him to write down what he remembered about Grace and me. He was only three at the time we packed up and left the The Old School House with his help.

It's very hard because I was so little. I can remember going there when I was very little, Grace looked lovely. She was old and had straight silver hair to her shoulders with curly ends. If you got really hot temperatures she could talk. I remember her saying a couple of words to me but I can't remember what they were.

Ray was kind with grey silver hair like Grace's but a wee bit tangly. He liked taking Grace to all the warm places in the world. I know they've been to Peru and I think Africa because they gave me a picture of an elephant. We used to take them to the airport and get an ice cream and wave to them on the plane from the balcony at the top of the escalators. I used to have a mint-choc-chip ice cream and you used to have either a vanilla or a strawberry one.

They could only eat organic things and we used to do their shopping. They drank lots of water in bottles. I can remember a big greenhouse, wild red fruit growing behind the garage, the apple trees, and crawling through a hole in the hedge to get into the park next door [Lanton village hall] then I'd have organic shortbread and fruit juice with Grace in the garden. Ray did all the cooking and some housework.

Their house had lots and lots of ornaments, some weird horses [the Cloisonné ones from China], and bracelets in boxes. The garage was packed with stuff! There was no way they could get the car in a garage full of boxes so Ray sold it because Ray's boxes were full of his favourite things, and as the house was already full of boxes he had nowhere else to store them. Anyway the car had a flat battery so it was a good idea to sell it. That's about it really.

His mother, Jane, was also kind enough to write to me with her impressions of Grace and me during that period:

Not long after I married a man who changed into shorts the moment he finished work, regardless of the depth of snow and lack of electricity in our soon-to-be-renovated cottage, I spotted a Border collie, obviously powered by yo-yos, bouncing along the road, oblivious to the horizontal rain and howling gale. Behind the hound, emerging over the brow of the hill, came an elderly couple. The husband, also oblivious to nature's worst efforts, was wearing a waterproof top, wellies and fluorescent batik shorts that flapped around his knees. In that instant I knew I was doomed to married life with a man who would never ever feel the cold as he aged, and progress into a more sophisticated version of casual wear. But far, far worse was the thought that I would end up dressed in shorts just as the elderly lady was, as they strolled down the hill past our house to seek their messages in town. For someone who only leaves her thermal underwear off for about a week in high summer, the thought of exposing so much flesh was horrific.

Over the following months we progressed from nodding acquaintance to sitting around the kitchen table with tea and cake. Grace and Ray had arrived in our lives. Grace spoke little except to deliver astute comic one-liners on the level of Ray's achievement in his role as chief cook and bottle washer, and to share a golden memory of their children prompted by some action from our baby. During these moments her natural softness and glow took on an extra radiance, like cashmere mixed with silk. Ray with his twinkling eyes, fluffy moustache and wild unruly hair looked like a T. H. White creation – a man who could boast Merlin as his ancestor and who had the ability to defy convention and make folk question their values. Now, depending on your viewpoint, Ray could either be seen as a stubborn, eccentric man who not only dragged his poor wife all over the countryside but had the temerity to repeat this heinous behaviour all over the world; or as an enlightened individual, who paid no creed to the conventional treatment designated to people like Grace but instead maintained the intellectual roaming lifestyle established in their youth, which now included Ray acquiring some eclectic culinary and housekeeping skills. If, like me, your only experience of tofu has been a gastronomic disaster presented in a bowl of soy sauce, then you should try Ray's complete nutritional tofu flapjack-cum-cake with nuts and fruity bits – it too defies convention, but tastes truly wonderful.

John and I are considered by our families to be hoarders – a term inflicted with exasperation but received as a compliment. However, when we went to help tidy Ray's garage, we were confronted with a wall of boxes piled floor to ceiling, length and breadth. Upon opening the doors, we realised that we were in the presence of true professionals. Grace and Ray were hoarders of megalithic proportions, masters of their art, for you would not stuff a garage to the gunnels if your house was not already bursting at the seams.

We learned a lot about our friends that weekend as we unearthed treasures, some of monetary and sentimental value but all with a history attached, interspersed with an inordinate amount of carpet tiles. Ray would be telling us about their mobile art gallery and we'd find a box of carpet tiles. We would listen (still unwrapping, cataloguing, sorting out items to keep, items to auction to fund their next great adventure) to their children's achievements, after finding a box of toys (and another box of carpet tiles). We were carried away (on carpet tiles) with accounts of Grace's trips to acquire fine art from China and Russia when another box of carpet tiles loomed before us. I can tell you, Scheherazade has nothing on this boy.

After two days and four trips to the skip, our car heaving with carpet tiles, we began to see the light. Eventually, suspense and repetitive carpet-tile shifting syndrome made us extract the longed-for story from him. The eyes started twinkling and his moustache began twitching as if tickled by a crescendo of chuckles, as he stood on a piece of garage floor experiencing the first glimpse of sunshine to hit it for years. 'Oh those,' he replied glibly, relishing our enthusiasm for more tales. 'I got those to place around the garden to suppress the weeds while we're away!' And off he hopped to Grace, grinning from ear to ear, to show her some more memorabilia from their intriguing past.

When you can view your treasured heaps of stuff and recall every nuance of their acquisition with such love and joy, it must be very hard to accept their early departure to pastures new – especially when the one person you love, cherish and adore wakes up each morning slightly altered from the day before, when their memories of life, love, family and you are no longer shared and become no longer accessible to the outside world; you must look at that person and wonder, Am I still there? Do you still hold memories of me within your pretty head? Then, more than at any other time, it would seem appropriate to hang on to and cherish your joint collected heritage, taking comfort in the memories it triggers. But Ray has never shown any signs of floundering in the pit of depression. Life for them both is a continuing quest to be followed together, and so their 'treasures' were car-booted to fund the next great adventure, for there was no doubt that, away from our cold climate, Grace blossomed in the heat. Photographs of her in the Galapagos Islands have a spark that is absent when she is home in the Borders.

One exception to this was the warm summer when our daughter was born. I had finished trimming Grace's hair in their conservatory and was just melting in my shoes when she started talking about our baby. I was flabbergasted. I hadn't heard her speak, let alone ask a simple question and make observations, for months. It was fantastic and worth getting heat stroke for. Robert was now three and fully appreciated this momentous event by organising a party – fruit juice, shortbread and a game of peek-a-boo, which was conducted solely between him and Grace, leaving Ray, wee Elaine and me as onlookers.

There are many more memories I could tell you, but

running through them all is the memory of the care and love and Ray's relentless research into vitamins that has kept the essence of Grace burning bright and strong, long after that of her peers has been extinguished.

I warn you now: Ray and Grace's lifestyle is contagious. Our son recalls their house as an Aladdin's cave, the garage fantastic, and sub-consciously feels compelled to fill his room, our room, and the living room with treasure acquired from car boots, table-top sales and other sources – and it's not all toys, but objects that 'will be collectable one day'. His younger sister is displaying the same symptoms. They both feel that people of any age, any ability, can do anything if they set their minds to it. (That's me they pencilled in for trekking in the Himalayas as an octogenarian clad in industrial-strength thermal underwear!) John and I know that whatever the future holds for us, we will know which path to follow – it's the one signposted 'Grace and Ray woz 'ere'. And paved with carpet tiles!

Stupid decision or not, I had made it. I sold the house in Lanton, and everything in it, put the money in the bank and we set off back to Peru. I hadn't realised how much junk we had built up over the years until I started trying to sort it out, and I was pleased to see it go. None of it was any use to Grace any more since it triggered no memories, and I had enough to think about organising the present without dwelling on the past. I'd got used to travelling light and I liked the idea of not having a house full of stuff any more, cutting things down to the minimum. Watching Grace had taught me that cluttering your life with memories is pointless and merely gets in the way of enjoying the present moment.

Grace had built up a library of books over the years, which I gave to Lanton village hall, along with the shelving needed to hold it. There were all the beautifully bound books from the Folio Society, and the big coffee-table *Readers Digest* books on all the important cultures of the world. Grace didn't always read her books cover to cover, but believed they should be opened occasionally and a few pages savoured, as if keeping them alive. She had books on all the subjects that had caught her attention over the years, from Hare Krishna to transcendental meditation.

My plan was to head for a market town called Cajamarca, nearly 3,000 metres up in the Andes, where Pizarro, the Spanish conquistador, ambushed and executed Atahualpa, the Inca ruler in 1533, going on to subdue the whole Inca empire and found the city of Lima. We'd been there before, and I knew that Grace enjoyed the spa baths that were filled from the thermal springs. We could get in for about a dollar, sitting amongst the local families, swishing our feet around in the water. After bathing we would sit in the floral garden and breathe the fumes and steam from the springs, have a picnic, get back to the hotel for a siesta and then go out to a noisy restaurant filled with Peruvian families or old men, where the food would be good and cheap. Sometimes musicians would wander around the diners as darkness fell, entertaining them with singing and music.

We stayed at the Cajamarca Hotel, a lovely Spanish-style

building with overhanging beams, in a room on the ground floor with its own shower and toilet. When we arrived I thought we could stay there for a couple of months, while we worked out how to become permanent residents in the country. But, even in paradise, reality has a habit of catching up with you.

What I didn't realise was that things were going to become far more difficult very quickly as Grace's condition declined, and that a country like Peru was not as well set up to provide help as you might hope. She had started to have epileptic fits about once a month, and there were no social services we could turn to for special equipment or nursing help. When we needed a wheelchair in Lima, for instance, the only one I was able to get hold of fell to pieces almost immediately, leaving us stranded. Getting hold of the supplements and vitamins Grace needed became a long, drawn-out process, reliant on a postal system that was less than regular, and then there were customs charges on top.

I was becoming less and less able to cope with Grace's needs. When she fell in the shower one day I had to call for a mobile medical service to come and put a couple of stitches into her head where she had cut it on the floor. Usually I was in time to catch her when she fell, but it was becoming more difficult as her movements became ever less predictable.

The fact that she was no longer able to speak or communicate at all meant that I really could never leave her side unless I could be confident she was fast asleep and would remain so for some hours. Things were becoming too hard. I realised I would have to accept defeat on the idea of moving to Peru, and admit that I needed the support of the British welfare system. It was a sad realisation, but I felt I had given the disease a good run for its money before having to accept that I needed assistance. There was no shame in admitting that I had dreamed one dream too many and overstepped what could actually be achieved. We started the long journey back to England with no idea what might lie in store for us next, now that our home in Lanton was gone, along with all our possessions.

CHAPTER ELEVEN

THE FINAL MONTHS

What will survive of us is love.

PHILIP LARKIN

It was only in the last few months that caring for Grace became too demanding to be fun. In the years leading up to the end I had enjoyed every minute of looking after her, being with her and loving her.

I realised that I had made a mistake thinking we could move away to South America permanently, but that didn't have to be a problem. We had always been happy together in Britain, and we would be again. I have always been too much of a dreamer, and too impulsive. I remember once, many years before, when I had the travelling gallery, there was a petrol shortage in the country and I thought there was a danger I might not be able to get enough fuel to ply my trade. On a whim I went out and bought an old horse-drawn gig which was delivered to the house. A surprised Grace answered the front door to be greeted by a man who simply said, 'Gig?'

It was a beautiful thing, but even if the fuel had run out, and even if I'd owned a horse, it would have been far too small to carry any paintings around in. I had simply wanted to own it because it was so beautiful, and I had looked for an excuse to justify my purchase. In the end it sat in the garage until I needed the space for something else and had to sell it. I think I did make a profit on the deal, but that was more by luck than judgement.

When we arrived back in Britain with no home, I knew that I needed to get as much help as I could from other members of the family. I contacted Grace's relations in Scotland, including Anne, but they didn't want anything to do with us by then. I guess they thought that I had brought the situation on myself, which was quite true, and should therefore sort it out myself. I could understand their exasperation, but I was hurt that they didn't even seem to want to see us.

I decided we should return to Peterborough, the city where I had started my life and where both my brothers were still living. Kenneth, my middle son, picked us up at the airport and drove us to a hotel in the city centre. The next day I went round to see the remaining family members. My older brother, Bill, didn't answer the door to me, but Reg and his wife were very kind, driving us around and helping me to organise a comfortable new life for Grace.

Bill would later be very sweet to our other son, Clifford, helping him out with a car when he needed one, and other things, but neither Bill nor Clifford seemed to want anything to do with me and Grace. Perhaps it was harder for other people to see her in those last months than it was for me. The changes had all been so gradual to me that she had never stopped being the same woman I had fallen in love with nearly half a century before. To anyone who had not seen her for a while the decline would have been dramatic and undoubtedly upsetting.

I still had what was left of the money from the sale of the house in Lanton, and I managed to find a small modern bungalow on a large estate on the outskirts of the city. We settled in, having just enough money left over to buy some basic pieces of new furniture to replace everything that we'd sold just a few months before. The bungalow had a pleasant little garden, where some mature shrubs and small trees allowed Grace to sit in privacy and watch the birds when it was warm enough, and where I could practise my Taikwondo, a martial art using the hands and feet which I had taken up many years before when it first arrived in Glasgow, partly to keep fit with the punching, kicking and blocking, and partly in case I ever needed some form of self-defence.

I had taken the boys to the classes as well. It was something we did together. There was a saying, which the instructors taught us: 'Don't take knives. Don't take guns. Take kwondo.' Sadly it wasn't enough to make Christopher feel safe from his imagined persecutors. I've never been physically attacked anywhere I've gone in the world (although I have, in common with many tourists, had my bag stolen) and I think that is a lot to do with giving the appearance of being confident and unafraid, which is what mastery of a martial art gives you. If you feel you can defend yourself then your body language will convey that message to others. It was never supposed to be an aggressive sport; the chant that we did at every class was that Taikwondo was 'for self-defence and for the defence of the weak'.

Once we were back in Peterborough, the local authority was very good at giving us devices that made it possible for me to continue caring for Grace at home, like ramps over all the steps to allow easy wheelchair access. As well as the various contraptions in the bathroom, such as a shower-and-toilet chair with a harness to maintain body and chest position for safe breathing, there was also an electric hoist over the bed to help me get her in and out and into the toilet chair, and a manual hoist in the living room so that I could transfer her to her Kirton adjustable armchair, which helped her correct postural problems and allowed me to feed her safely.

We were also able to get a comfortable, padded Netti medical wheelchair for outdoor use. Made in Norway, it gave a good range of positions for comfort and support. This could be provided with additional equipment for head and arm support, adjustable leg support and could be adapted for other medical uses. A tray could be fitted to confine the arms and as a base for feeding when we were travelling.

And so Grace's days fell into another steady routine. At eight o'clock I would get her up, wheel her into the shower to wash her and play. By nine we would be ready to return to bed for a fresh nappy and some physiotherapy. I would then dress her. By ten thirty I would have pushed her through to the conservatory, where I would give her half a cup of spring water and 2,000µg B12, leaving her to listen to music while I prepared breakfast. At about eleven I would give her organic fruit mashed up, organic cereals, juice and the following: 4,000mg vitamin C with bioflavonoids, 250mg vitamin B6, 1000 IU vitamin E, 800µg folic acid, 500mg niacin, 200µg selenium, 45mg elemental zinc, one Solgar advanced carotenoid complex and one Solgar VM 75 multivitamin with minerals.

By half past twelve Grace was ready to be wheeled back to the bathroom, where I would strap her to the toilet. She would sit there, quite happily, for an hour or so because I felt it was important that she had a good bowel movement. Sometimes I would use this opportunity to take a nap if I had had a disturbed night.

At two we would be ready for our slow walk around the cul-de-sac, or wherever I pushed the wheelchair to, and then back home for our main meal, which would still consist of oily fish three days a week, and organic bacon, eggs and cheese on the others, plus lots of organic vegetables and potatoes. For dessert I would produce fruit with cream, ice cream or yoghurt, or cake, most of which would be organic as well. We would drink Typhoo tea with milk and sugar. Since neither of us had many of our own teeth left by then, most of our food was minced, mashed or cut up small enough to swallow without too much chewing.

At six in the evening I would strap Grace to the toilet again and give her another fresh nappy, clean her teeth with floss and a soft brush, and wash her face without using soap. By eight we were ready to go to bed, with a Beethoven symphony playing in the background and three packs of nappies on either side of Grace to keep her protected if she kicked out, which she often did. The cot sides that I had taken to attaching to the bed stopped her from falling out. Much like the cot sides designed for children, I found these invaluable. I believe the kicking was a way for her to relieve the tensions that built up in her muscles from so much inactivity. Grace would always drop off right away. At one o'clock in the morning I would change her nappy, and at odd times of the night I would ensure her bedclothes were settled and comfortable. By that time she was still able to raise her head a little.

Many years before, she had gone through these same rituals with the boys in Scotland, making sure they were safe and comfortable in their makeshift cots at night, ensuring that they had the right amounts of food at the right times, and that they were always clean and comfortable. It was as if her life clock was running backwards at a terrible speed, carrying her back towards the oblivion from which we all emerge.

Once a week I would ring Dial-a-Ride, who would send round a minibus that was equipped to take the wheelchair, and we would set off into town to do our shopping in the Queensgate Centre, and stop off at the College Arms for a meal, where I would enjoy a Guinness and Grace would have a juice.

I put on an exhibition at the Great Northern Hotel of photographs, stories, poems and articles about Grace's life, to which the local press gave quite a bit of coverage. I was proud of her and liked people to know about her and about how well she had responded to the way her illness had been treated.

It might have been better if I had let them take her in for a few days' respite care now and then, to give us both a break. I did it once, when I wanted to go to a conference on Alzheimer's at Loughborough University, and it was very nice to be relieved of the responsibility for a few days. Apart from the one time I had tried it before, many years earlier, this was the first time we had been apart for more than an hour or two in ten years. But I wouldn't have wanted to be without her in the years before.

She benefited from the respite as well because there were other patients and nurses buzzing around, which was stimulating for her; and, as she no longer recognised me, she didn't know I wasn't there. It was a particularly nice place, which a social worker had found for me when I said I wanted to get away. I knew I was very lucky to have found it – most places that look after the old and infirm are not as pleasant as that.

I'm certain that Grace never lost her awareness of human kindness or the need to love and be loved. When people did take the trouble to talk to her or communicate with her, she always responded with joy, even when she had no idea who they were or what they were saying.

Things were getting increasingly difficult at home because

she was having trouble swallowing her food. I knew that it wasn't going to be long before she was going to have to go into a hospital and be fed through a tube. I was holding out against that for as long as possible, coaxing the puréed food down her throat whenever I could, but I was aware I wouldn't be able to do it for much longer.

Even then I still wanted to travel rather than sit around the house all day. I realised that I was going to have to be a little less ambitious than in the past and find a destination that was equipped for wheelchairs. I discovered a hotel in Tenerife that could supply everything, including a bed with a cot side and a hoist, so that I would be able to lift her in and out easily. I could see no reason why we couldn't spend some weeks down there, in the warm, living exactly as we did at home, and made the booking. Unfortunately, Grace was not able to make that final journey.

CHAPTER TWELVE

THE END

Why fear death? It is the most
beautiful adventure in life.

*LAST WORDS OF CHARLES FROHMAN BEFORE
DROWNING IN THE LUSITANIA*

I never thought about Grace dying. When it did happen I was shocked, even though I knew that she would eventually die of the complications arising from her Alzheimer's, and even though I realised that we couldn't go on much longer together. I had blocked out the idea of her actually going because I didn't want to imagine my life without her there.

All through the summer of 2002 it was becoming increasingly difficult to feed her, and she was growing weak as a result, not really having taken any sustenance for a week or more. I called the doctor and he came out to see her. His advice was to make her comfortable and leave her to die. He thought that would be the kindest thing, and I understood why he said it. I even agreed to do as he suggested, but once he had gone I realised it was impossible. I had been fighting for so long to keep her alive, I couldn't just sit by and let her die. I still loved her and I wanted to be with her. He was going away on holiday and I didn't want to wait until he got back, so I rang the hospital the next day and asked for help. They took her in, and I would sit beside her bed from eight in the morning until seven each evening, nursing her just as I would do at home. They managed to build her strength enough for me to bring her back to the bungalow again after a few weeks.

Every day I would still take her out in the wheelchair, just as I had when she was able to walk with me. When we had reached somewhere pleasant I would get her to stand up, holding both her hands and walking backwards in front of her as she shuffled forward a few steps, just as much as she could manage without falling. There was a nice walk behind the bungalow along a path, which went through an avenue of giant redwoods to a big old house that had been turned into a luxury hotel. We'd gone into the hotel once to look around the big hall and the staff had been preparing for a wedding. A lady was setting up her harp to play to the guests, and she invited us to stay and listen to her practise. It was a lovely moment, listening to that gentle, celestial music in such beautiful surroundings with the sun shining down on to the gardens outside.

The autumn passed and it was on 21 December, when we were out beneath the giant redwoods, that I noticed Grace had a bit of a cough. The path was thick with leaves, making it difficult to push the chair, and so I'd taken a broom out with us and was doing some sweeping as she watched, all wrapped up against the cold.

The next day was a Sunday, and our routine was as normal, with an early morning shower but I noticed she was still coughing. I knew that she was vulnerable to infections because of the disease, and so I called the doctor at about ten. He came out an hour later and said she should have some antibiotics, which I already had in the house from some previous problem. Because of her swallowing difficulties it was hard to get even a spoonful of medicine into her, but I persevered. The swallowing was becoming an increasing problem, often preventing me from being able to get her to take the tablets and supplements that I believe had been helping her to fight infections in the previous years.

She didn't want any lunch, and I didn't think I should take her out in the cold until she had fought off the infection, so I settled her down in her chair in the corner of the conservatory and set the music playing on the radio. I then went into the adjoining sitting room to have a little sleep on the sofa. I often took afternoon naps, when I could, because the nights were always interrupted by nappy changes and looking after Grace all day made me tired. The sofa was only about ten feet away from the chair, so I was confident I would wake up if she was in any sort of distress. Normally she would doze off as well if she was sitting comfortably in the warm.

I fell into a deep sleep and woke up about three hours later. It was dark outside and silent in the conservatory apart from the music, which was still playing quietly. Grace seemed to be peaceful. I went through to see if she needed anything. I thought I would try to get her to swallow some more of the medicine while she was relaxed, but I couldn't get her to open her mouth and I realised she had passed away.

Despite everything I was surprised by the suddenness with which the end had come, and all I wanted was for her to be alive still.

You'd think that death would be dramatic in some way, but it is quite the opposite. The house was just dark and quiet, and there was nothing for me to do once I'd called the doctor. He came and signed a death certificate, so there didn't have to be a post-mortem, and the undertakers came from the Co-op, kindly letting me say goodbye to her before they took her off to the mortuary to dress her for the grave.

Then the house was empty, and there was nothing for me to do but go to bed on my own. I felt as bereft as I had in the days when we first met at the nurses' home and she used to have to leave my room after making love. Just as I had then written poems to her to make it feel like she was still with me, I sat down now and wrote a eulogy for her funeral. The ceremony was to be on 3 January.

Kenneth, realising how devastated I was by the sudden bereavement, drove all the way up from London to collect me and take me down to his home in Wimbledon for Christmas with his family. It was a gesture of enormous kindness and thoughtfulness. I think I would have found it very hard to be alone in the bungalow in the first few days after she was gone, seeing her empty bed and her empty chair, having the long hours of each day stretching out, empty until I had thought of new ways to fill them with something other than sadness. It gave me time to collect my thoughts and prepare myself for the final stage of the process.

Years before, when Grace was still in full possession of her faculties, we had agreed that we both wanted green burials. We wanted cardboard coffins because the idea of cutting down beautiful trees just to bury them in the ground or burn them seemed criminal. We both believed that death should be a natural thing. Just as the body of a bird or rabbit that dies in the wild is quickly absorbed into the earth and eaten by insects or predators, we felt that we too should provide a feast for the worms.

I didn't like the idea of standing around in a graveyard, saying goodbye to Grace. I always hated the atmosphere of those places, with the artificial crunch of the neat gravel paths and the sinister stones looming up all around. A green burial takes place in a field, surrounded by trees.

Grace's coffin was actually made of bamboo, a sustainable crop that can be harvested twice a year with no damage to the environment, and the only sign that the burial ground is not a normal field is the plaques, inset in the ground with simple messages of people's names and the dates of their lives. The coffin was nicely lined and trimmed, and Grace looked lovely lying in it.

The mourners, and the funeral officials, were all asked to

attend in casual clothes and just to say a few words. I had the eulogy I had written to her the moment she had gone in my pocket. Only two of her children, Kenneth and Anne, were there. It didn't seem worth contacting Christopher; I don't think the news would have meant anything to him, and I don't know what happened to Clifford. It was cold and there was a light rain falling, but bad weather had never bothered Grace and me.

This book is really an extended version of my eulogy to Grace. It ended like this:

'Grace was the only girl I ever loved. I have never met a person so wonderful, so kind and gentle, never saying a bad word about anyone – a real peace lover.'

I promised Grace I would treat the writing of this book with the greatest urgency, answering no letters and taking part in no other activity until it is finished. The world has lost a truly great person.

I love you, Grace.

EPILOGUE: THE GREAT VITAMIN DEBATE

Alzheimer's affects half a million people in Britain, and that figure is expected to grow by fifty per cent over the next twenty years. It has been known for several centuries that diet could intimately affect mental health, so this is not just some passing fad. In 1740 James Lind, a naval surgeon, discovered that sailors went mad when they were deprived of fresh vegetables. As soon as he put them back on a balanced diet they were immediately cured. In the intervening quarter of a millennium western man has been so bedazzled by the achievements and claims of scientists that we have been distracted from some of the most basic truths. We have all heard the cliché 'you are what you eat', but all too often we forget that this is true for our minds as well as our bodies.

Case histories that prove the connection between nutrition

and mental health abound. There was once a common disease called pellagra, which caused dementia and other symptoms. As soon as it was discovered that it was caused by a deficiency of vitamin B3, the disease was wiped out. It has also been known for a long time that alcoholics require large doses of vitamins to rid themselves of the mental symptoms associated with their addiction, and that babies suffering severe mental disturbance can often be cured with zinc supplements.

When I read an article by Joe Hattersley which claimed that dog food is upgraded every three years to a new nutritional high, that the recommended daily allowances for dogs were better researched and higher than those for people, and that veterinary nutrition was fifty years ahead of human nutrition, I thought I would do some investigating of my own. He also claimed that mineral supplements for people don't provide nearly as many necessary minerals as the supplements routinely given to both dogs and farm animals.

I popped into the local supermarket and bought a variety of pet foods, taking them home to study. Admittedly, most of it is processed gunk. Dogs are given meat 'derivatives', and I'm frightened even to think what that might mean. The point was that, added into this stodgy gloop which passes for meat, the manufacturers had pumped extremely high doses of vitamins. On a can of brand-name dog food, for instance, I discovered that it provided 1,500 IU of vitamin A for every kilogram, or about 700 IU per can, which is the daily meal for your average dachshund. In addition, it contained 70mg of vitamin D in each can, 40mg of vitamin E and 1mg of copper.

There was a complete complement of vitamins and minerals.

If you translate those levels up from a 5kg dog to a 58kg human such as myself, I should have 8,120 IU of vitamin A in my food before I even get near my supplements, 812mg of vitamin D and 464mg of vitamin E. Just looking at this can alone I could see that my hypothetical dachshund would be getting higher nutrients than the European Parliament wanted to give any single member of the population of Europe under their new vitamin laws.

I then examined a dried hard tack of lamb, rice, corn and fish meat intended for cats, and found one of the healthiest of superfoods: brewer's yeast. It also included 12,000 IU per kg of vitamin A and a whopping 955 IU per kg of vitamin E.

Working my way on down the size scale I found that hamster food contained 14,000 IU of vitamin A per kg, 2,000 IU of vitamin D3 and 60mg of vitamin E. Even the seeds and cereals given to budgerigars contained iodine and calcium and more vitamins per kg than the EU believe is safe for humans. The animals' supplements also leave ours in the dust, including chromium and vanadium to help eliminate animal diabetes. No law requires those trace minerals to be present in human food. In fact, at the time of writing, the Food Supplements Directive is planning to ban them in human supplements. So, unpalatable as the thought may be, we might actually be better off eating pet food.

There are so many different theories, old wives' tales and nuggets of misinformation circulating about what we should and shouldn't eat that it's not surprising that many people simply give up trying to work out what would be the best path for them. For many years it has been believed that fats and cholesterol cause heart disease. In fact, they are simply indications that something is awry, metabolically speaking, usually due to a deficiency of the nutrients we need to run at full throttle. Cholesterol only got the blame because of incorrectly interpreted animal research – yet another good reason never to rely on information from animal research when you are looking for answers in humans.

Dr John Mansfield, a panel member of *What Doctors Don't Tell You*, argues that heart disease began the moment we started industrialising food, refining, processing and stripping it of heart-protective nutrients like the B vitamins, chromium and magnesium. It may also have something to do with eating more protein, particularly animal protein, than our bodies can efficiently process. Mansfield notes that, while the amount of fat in our diets has not increased significantly over the past century, refined sucrose intake has increased by over 1,000 per cent. This alone would suggest that a high-sugar and processed-carbohydrate diet, rather than one high in cholesterol and fat, is the major culprit in heart disease.

If all the renegade heart researchers are even half right, the implications are enormous, causing no less than a revolution in the way we understand and treat coronary artery disease, and toppling the orthodox approaches to heart-disease treatment with their reliance on dangerous procedures such as bypass surgery, temporary solutions like angioplasty, or the host of inhibitors and blockers, thinners and reducers that the drug companies have come up with to suppress the symptoms. It could also mean the end of the lucrative low-fat and low-cholesterol food industry, which results in yet more plastic food posing as a healthy option. Most of all it makes the solution to heart disease amazingly simple. All we've got to do to cut the risks of heart attacks is eat good, wholesome food and take a few vitamins.

One of the barriers to these ideas catching on is that it would put a lot of people out of business. Compared with the thousands of pounds that a typical bypass costs, Dr Mansfield reckons that getting all the tests he deems necessary to check your homocysteine and all your vitamin and mineral levels would cost, at most, £133. Instead of a cocktail of expensive heart drugs, patients could take a few inexpensive supplements to avoid illness.

It appears that high levels of homocysteine, with shrinkage of the brain in middle age, can lead later to Alzheimer's, with up to fifteen per cent of all dementia cases being caused this way. Homocysteine has an effect on the brain decades before people develop obvious signs of Alzheimer's. There is already strong evidence linking it with heart disease, deep-vein thrombosis and strokes. An individual can lower homocysteine by taking folic acid.

MRI scans of more than 1,000 apparently healthy people aged between fifty and seventy showed that those who had higher homocysteine levels six or eight years before had smaller brain volumes and performed less well in tests. These results added to previous findings suggesting that homocysteine may play an important part in mental as well as physical ageing. Either homocysteine produces changes in the arteries, affecting the brain, or there is a toxic effect.

Homocysteine is a substance that we make in our bodies when we digest any kind of animal protein and some vegetables. Various research groups have reached the conclusion that high levels of homocysteine in the blood may be linked to disorders of, or damage to, blood vessels, and that it can be affected by vitamins B6, B12 and folate to lessen the chances of Alzheimer's or dementia. Low levels of these substances lead to a rise of homocysteine in the blood because the enzymes that are supposed to reduce levels of homocysteine require these vitamins to function effectively.

If homocysteine can damage blood vessels, including those to the brain, it could cause changes in memory and mental function. Some scientists believe that it could be said to poison brain cells. Researchers have studied the levels of homocysteine in the blood of Alzheimer's sufferers, as well as those with vascular dementia (a disease caused by abnormalities in the blood vessels, but not affecting the brain in the same way as Alzheimer's) and stroke sufferers. They then recorded the levels of B vitamins and folate to see if it was possible to assess a risk factor for blood vessel or heart problems. The results showed that the levels of homocysteine were higher in the blood of patients in all the disease groups, compared with the controls, concluding that 'mildly elevated homocysteine levels may therefore significantly increase the risk of vascular dementia, Alzheimer's and stroke'. They also ruled out the possibility that variations in a gene linked to homocysteine metabolism could be responsible for the raised levels and increased dementia risk, although they did identify one variant of the gene that was linked to an increased risk of vascular dementia and possibly to the development of dementia that some people develop after a stroke. A conclusion reached from the study was that folate or vitamin B12 supplements could be useful to elderly people, particularly those at raised risk of blood vessel disease or dementia.

Diet is not the entire story of heart health, any more than it is the single solution to any other medical problem. For example, it is well documented that many people develop heart disease and die from loneliness – literally dying of a broken heart. But diet is certainly one of the most important factors, if not the most important.

Heart disease is not, therefore, a problem of abundance, as we have been led to believe in the past, but one of scarcity, a symptom of deficiency, not greed. Heart disease patients following low-fat diets are probably only making matters worse. Rather than starving ourselves of foods vital to our health, we need to eat more heartily, nutritionally speaking, than we have for a long time

Vitamin deficiency is particularly common among the old, and it seems highly likely that increasing the intake of B vitamins will help prevent Alzheimer's and other forms of dementia. B6, B12 and folate are of particular importance.

Experts now recommend 2–5mg of folic acid and a similar dose of vitamin B12 daily. Vitamin B12, also known as cobalamin, is bound to the protein in food and helps maintain healthy nerve cells and red blood cells. It is also needed to manufacture DNA, the genetic material that exists in all cells. Hydrochloric acid in the stomach releases B12 from protein during digestion and, once released, it combines with a substance called intrinsic factor and then becomes absorbed into the bloodstream. B12 is naturally found in animal foods including fish, milk and milk products, eggs, meat and poultry, and most fortified breakfast cereals also provide an excellent source, which is particularly useful for vegetarians.

Many still argue that if we eat a balanced diet we shouldn't need any supplements. But how many of us are able to eat a balanced diet? Even if we think that we are, what do we know of the quality of that which we are eating? Bad soil management and intensive farm methods have undoubtedly lowered the quality of much of the food in the shops. In 1992 the Earth Summit in Rio stated that the average farm soils in America were eighty per cent depleted of minerals, compared to a worldwide depletion of seventy-five per cent. There may be more food on our plates and in our shops; our food may even look bigger and better than it used to; but it does not have the same nutritional value. Reports warning that this has been happening have been written since 1936. Farmers are under too much pressure to produce results, which means they cannot afford to use traditional methods for restoring fertility to the soil like cover crops, crop rotation and leaving fields to lie fallow. The soil becomes exhausted after a few years and the only way to revive it, or at least give the appearance of doing so, is with fertilisers containing nitrogen, phosphorus and potassium. The yields look good and the farmers get paid, but the minerals and vitamins are missing.

Between 1940 and 1999 carrots lost seventy-five per cent of their magnesium, forty-eight per cent of their calcium, forty-six per cent of their iron and seventy-five per cent of their copper. Broccoli and spring onions both lost seventy-five per cent of their calcium, and the figures were just as bad for every other kind of fruit and vegetable. To get the same amount of copper as one tomato would have given you in 1940, you would now need to eat at least ten; to get the same amount of iron as you would have got from one of those oranges I was given in Haifa all those years ago, you would now have to eat three or more.

By putting only sodium, phosphorus and potassium into the soil we have changed the ratios between the minerals in the food we grow. In 1940 there was a two-to-one ratio between phosphorous and calcium, now it is one-to-one. Swedes, for instance, now contain 110 per cent of the phosphorous they once did. These changes are bound to have an effect on the bodies into which they are introduced.

The non-organic food most of us are eating is like the dog food, but without the supplements. It may be well packaged and attractive to the eye, but it is poor quality. High doses of supplements are not a luxury for those who are obsessed with their own health; they are crucial for the maintenance of basic good health in everyone.

Most adults need to supplement their food with 500mg of calcium citrate, lactate or gluconate, 200–400mg of magnesium citrate, gluconate or chelates, 10mg of any sort of iron except sulphates, 15–30mg of zinc (citrate, gluconate or chelate), 100μg of chromium, up to 200mg of selenium, 500μg of iodine, 2–3mg of copper, 300–600mg of potassium, 3mg of boron and 5–25mg of manganese.

It is important to get yourself tested so that you know what deficiencies you have, so that you can take steps to counteract them. Recommended daily allowances (RDAs) can't always be relied on: they are usually only the minimum quantity of nutrient required to maintain metabolic balance or to prevent disease due to vitamin deficiency. Different cultural groups, individual requirements, daily diets or biochemical individuality mean that everyone requires different doses to achieve different effects.

It is important not to supplement indiscriminately. More isn't always better and some vitamins, such as A and E, can actually become toxic if you take too much. It may also be that your body is sufficiently biochemically efficient not to need everything that some nutrients provide. It's also possible that your stomach acid is not strong enough to absorb some pills. Your ability to assimilate will depend on a number of different factors including your genetic disposition, the state of your health and your age.

It is always a good idea to take extra minerals such as magnesium and zinc – none of us get enough of them. Take minerals such as citrates, fumarates, gluconates, amino acid chelates, aspartates or picolinates and avoid metallic or inorganic forms of minerals such as oyster shell, egg shell and the inorganic iron that pollutes all processed foods. If the pH (acid/base) balance is not right, calcium supplements are likely to be excreted.

Make sure your diet contains sufficient fat-soluble vitamins and nutrients, which include vitamins E, A and D, plus the essential fatty acids. You will get one portion of vitamin D from sunlight on your skin, but you also need to consume sea foods, especially fatty fish such as herring and salmon, animal organs like liver, and dairy products such as cheese and butter. If you are not getting all these then you need to supplement them.

Vitamin C, beta-carotene and vitamin E are all important antioxidants, and their decline in natural foods is a problem. They protect us against the free radicals that our bodies generate in our normal metabolism and from the many toxins we encounter in the environment. They also protect us from the many problems that we normally associate with ageing. Men with the lowest intake of vitamin C, for instance, have a sixty-two per cent increased risk of cancer and fifty-seven per cent increased chance of dying prematurely from any cause.

Most animals and plants synthesise their own vitamin C, with humans being one of the few exceptions, having lost the ability around a million years ago. We are missing one of the six enzymes needed for converting glucose to Vitamin C and need to get it from our diet. An unstressed animal, depending on its size, manufactures between five and fifteen grams of the vitamin a day. When under stress they will double that production level.

Because glucose and vitamin C are similar structurally, it is possible that some of the sugar cravings we all experience from time to time actually indicate a need for vitamin C. The vitamin provides many important functions including cell repair and division, energy production and antioxidant effects which neutralise toxins. Most of us eat too few foods containing vitamin C, and at the same time amounts of the vitamin available to us naturally have decreased due to premature food harvesting, artificial ripening and food processing.

Small doses of vitamin C (1g or less) seem to have little effect on any condition. Large doses of 20–200g per day, however, can bring about significant positive changes, shortening the courses of diseases. Almost all conditions, acute or chronic, can have shortened courses, and patients respond favourably. Even doses of up to 300g per day, taken intravenously, seem to have no problematic side effects.

Vitamin C is probably the best anti-viral agent in existence, which is why so many people recommend it for the fight against colds, and why it is recommended in cases of chronic viral illness such as hepatitis, mononucleosis, lupus and AIDS. It also strengthens the immune system.

It is better to take vitamin C in the mixed ascorbic buffered salt form rather than the ascorbic acid form. The neutral pH of the salts is preferable to the acidic form as it's much better tolerated in large doses, and also serves as a vehicle for useful calcium, magnesium and potassium. It needs to be taken only to a level that the bowels can tolerate so as not to create gas, cramps or diarrhoea. This can happen when the absorptive tissues become saturated so that no more ascorbate can be absorbed. Increased peristalsis moves digestive products through the gut more quickly. It can also create uncomfortable gas. These reactions may be because the body has been so depleted of vitamin C in the past that when it comes it gives the intestine the strength to function again. Alternatively it may be the dying off of organisms that do not belong in the gut, or it might indicate a deficiency of the nutrients L-glutathione or bioflavonoid and quercetin, which all assist vitamin C uptake and metabolism.

It may take several weeks to achieve bowel tolerance, and if you want to stop ascorbate for any reason you must do so gradually. It's important, however, to push to bowel tolerance since many helpful things happen at saturation level. Doses of 50–200g per day are usual for immune dysfunctions like cancer, chronic viral and bacterial infections and other serious inflammatory or auto-immune diseases. If appropriate doses of vitamin C are taken through life it will charge up the cellular electron pool, promoting cellular healing and metabolism, purging the body of foreign invaders and providing a base on which to build health. During periods of stress or illness much more can be taken than at other times.

There are many who believe that lowered attention spans and increasing behavioural problems can all be traced back to soil depletion and the increasing scarcity of the vitamins, minerals and amino acids that our brains require to produce neurotransmitters and other crucial brain compounds.

Tests on *Ginkgo biloba* have suggested that it can improve memory and overall function for people with Alzheimer's. It is an extract from the leaves of the ginkgo or maidenhair tree, and it has been used for medical purposes for 5,000 years. The Alzheimer's Society and the Cochrane Collaboration, an international organisation reviewing health-care interventions, have published a comprehensive review on its use for the treatment of dementia, identifying thirty-three previous clinical trials and concluding that it appears to be safe to use with no excessive side effects compared with a placebo. Overall there is promising evidence of improvement in cognition and function associated with ginkgo.

In my view the recommended daily allowances of vitamins and minerals do not greatly help. I believe that only mega doses can succeed in the promotion and maintenance of good health. The following is a list of daily supplements that Grace and I found beneficial:

520mg *Ginkgo biloba*
250mg vitamin B6
200ug chromium picolinate
45mg elemental zinc
800ug folic acid
4,000mg vitamin C with bioflavonoids
200ug selenium

1,000 IU vitamin E

Solgar advanced carotenoid complex

essential fatty acids

green vegetables

Solgar VM 75 multivitamin with minerals

A POEM TO MY BEAUTIFUL GRACE

Oft in quiet meditation,
I think of you, this separation.
What I can do, my only part,
To win your love and take your heart?

Take your hand and lift our wings
Into the sky and better things,
Gliding softly o'er the clouds,
To leave behind the noise and crowds.

Right across the plainest lands,
Sighting oft the golden sands,
Waves and horses on the shores,
Beating 'gainst the rocky doors.

Till we reach the lochs and glens
Matchless, pure, ne'er caught by lens,
To Mendelssohn and 'Fingal's Cave',
Where we can rest amidst the wave.

But in your arms, I wonder whether,
Your mind is far away from here,
Midst the fragrance of the heather,
With someone else who must be dear.

Such response I long to hear,
But you're not here I'm sure.
No act, no touch, no simple gesture,
By word of mouth or slight of leg.

Perhaps in life I fill a purpose,
A gap in time conveniently,
Relieve the boredom of your days,
Perhaps to please in many ways.

So if I please, please let me know,
So in my heart, a germ you sow.
A little hope of love and pleasure,
Together we could know such leisure.

I do believe our aims are like,
Our love of life and all mankind.
Belief in rights, equality, justice.
Ambitions shared to make the world

A place where brothers will not fight.
Give all respect and each a right
To fullest life and joy and peace,
That happiness will never cease.

Appendix I

HELPFUL BOOKS

Hendler, Sheldon Saul *The Doctor's Vitamin and Mineral Encyclopedia* (Leopard Books, 1995)

Mindell, Earl *The Food Medicine Bible* (Souvenir Press, 1996)

Pfeiffer, Carl *Nutrition and Mental Illness* (Inner Traditions International, 1988)

Werback, Melvyn R *Nutritional Influences on Illness* (Keats Publishing, 1990)

Holford, Patrick *Say No To Cancer (The Optimum Nutrition Bible)* (Piatkus, 1999)

Courteney, Hazel *500 of the Most Important Health Tips You'll Ever Need* (Cico Books, 2001)

OTHER PUBLICATIONS

What Doctors Don't Tell You A monthly newsletter, edited by Lynne McTaggart and written in lay terms. It exposes the dangers of modern medicine. It offers up-to-the-minute proven scientific alternatives for diagnosing, preventing and treating many illnesses. *What Doctors Don't Tell You* has become my medical bible, and has helped me to take control of my own health. They also publish *Secrets of the Drug Industry* by Bryan Hubbard and *The Cancer Handbook*, both of which can be obtained from them. Their contact details are as follows:

What Doctors Don't Tell You
2 Salisbury Road
London SW19 4EZ
Tel: 020 8944 9555

The Lancet A weekly publication which covers all the latest medical news.

APPENDIX 2

USEFUL CONTACTS

The Alzheimer's Society
Gordon House
10 Greencoat Place
London SW1P 1PH
Telephone: 020 7306 0606
Fax: 020 7306 0808
E-mail: enquiries@alzheimers.org.uk
www.alzheimers.org

Alzheimer's Disease International
45–46 Lower Marsh
London SE1 7RG
Telelphone: 020 7620 3011
Fax: 020 7401 7351
E-mail: info@alz.co.uk
www.alz.co.uk

Alzheimer Scotland
22 Drumsheugh Gardens
Edinburgh EH3 7RN
Telephone: 0131 243 1453
Fax: 0131 243 1450
Helpline: 0800 808 3000
E-mail: alzheimer@alzscot.org
www.alzscot.org

Alzheimer Europe
www.alzheimer-europe.org

Age Concern
Age Concern England
Astral House
1268 London Road
London SW16 4ER
Information Line: 0800 009966
www.ageconcern.org.uk

Nutrition Associates Ltd
Galfres Ltd
Clifton House
Moregate
York
Tel: 01904 691 591

Accessible Travel and Leisure
Avionics House
Naas Lane
Quedgeley
Gloucester
GL2 2SN
Tel: 01452 729 739